ORAL MANIFESTATIONS OF PEDIATRIC CANCERS AND ITS MANAGEMENT

INTRA-ORAL CLINICAL FEATURES, COMPLICATIONS AND ITS MANAGEMENT

DR. ANKUR JAIN | DR. ARUNA RETHAN

Made with ♥ on the Notion Press Platform
www.notionpress.com

Contents

Introduction

The second most common cause of death in children is childhood cancer. It corresponds to a group of diseases characterized by the uncontrolled proliferation of atypical cells, which may occur anywhere in the body. The most common malignant neoplasms of childhood are the leukemias, central nervous system tumors, and the lymphomas.[1] Cancer cases are predicted to increase by 70% over the next two decades, according to the World Health Organisation. Cancer mortality is the top killer. Since the 2008 estimates, breast cancer incidence has increased by more than 20%, while mortality has increased by 14% and is the most frequently diagnosed cancer among women in 140 of 184 countries worldwide. After breast, colorectal, and lung cancers, cervical cancer is the fourth most common cancer affecting women worldwide.[2]

Years of intense biomedical research and billions of dollars spent in cancer research have increased the understanding of the underlying mechanisms of tumorigenesis and cancer biology. Although, despite advances in surgical and radiation treatments, chemotherapy continues to be an important therapeutic option for different malignancies, especially for the primary, advanced and metastatic tumors. However, the efficacy of chemotherapy is substantially limited by the intrinsic and acquired resistance of cancer cells to anticancer drugs.

Oral pathoses in children are often missed since obtaining detailed history and performing thorough clinical examination are more difficult in comparison with an adult. The belief of the clinician that children rarely suffer from oral pathoses further adds to lesser number of early diagnoses. Leukemia is the most common childhood cancer, accounting for 28% of cases, followed by brain and other nervous system tumors (26%). In adolescents, for example, brain and other nervous system tumors are most common (21%), greater than one-half of which are benign/borderline malignant, followed closely by lymphoma (20%). In addition, there are almost twice as many cases of Hodgkin as non-Hodgkin lymphoma, whereas among children, the reverse is true. Thyroid carcinoma and melanoma of the skin account for 11% and 4%, respectively, of cancers in adolescents, but only 2% and 1%, respectively, in children. The overall cancer incidence rate in children and adolescents has been increasing slightly (by 0.7% per year) since 1975 for reasons that remain unclear.[3]

Children undergoing cancer treatment have many symptoms and diseases that manifest themselves in an acute and chronic manner. Oral complications may be observed during chemotherapy and are important side effects that may directly affect the anticancer treatment. The medical treatment received by children with cancer is not aimed exclusively at treatment of the malignant disease but also involves preventing and managing the many possible complications of the treatment itself.[4]

Acute oral complications such as mucositis, xerostomia, bleeding, and infections occur three times more commonly in children than in adults.[5] Such complications can interrupt treatment. According to the American Academy of Pediatric Dentistry ([AAPD], 2008), "The most frequently documented source of sepsis in the immunosuppressed cancer patient is the mouth"[6]. Oral mucositis, gingivitis, herpetic stomatitis, and candidiasis are potential sources of systemic infections in patients receiving cancer chemotherapy.[7]

The entire population exhibits considerable amounts of variation in dental development. If an oncology professional is concerned about the eruption timing or sequence of a patient's dentition, a dental referral may be recommended for assessment. Dental lamina, the tissue from which teeth are derived, is evident from days 35–37 of embryonic life. Primary teeth begin calcification prior to birth, and calcification of permanent dentition commences with the first molar at about the time of birth. Dental development continues throughout childhood into adolescence; therefore, illness and medications throughout this time frame can be detrimental. Potential long-term and chronic effects of cancer treatment on the oral cavity in children include altered root development, enamel opacities, hypocalcification, periodontal issues, and higher caries rates.[8]

This dessertation is aimed at emphasizing the oral manifestations and management of cancers in pediatric patients.

CHAPTER I

PREVALENCE OF PEDIATRIC CANCERS IN INDIA

In 1975, The National Cancer Control Program was started. It focused on priorities like tobacco cessation and screening and the treatment of cervical and head and neck cancers, which constitute the major cancer burden in India.[9,10] Therefore the infrastructure and manpower were geared up to address these problems with a focus on establishing radiotherapy departments and machines. In India annually one million new cancers are diagnosed, 3% of these occur in children.[11] These 50,000 new pediatric cancers annually diagnosed in India comprise about 20% of all pediatric cancers in the world.[12] It is presumed that about 60% of the children with newly diagnosed cancers in India will succumb to the disease as opposed to only 10% of the children in the developed countries.[13]

The Institute of Medicine in 2001 defined six major domains for quality health-care, namely efficient, effective, equitable, safe, patient-centered, and timely.[14] (Table :1) analyzes each of these quality domains with regard to pediatric cancers in India.

TABLE: 1 Health Quality Domain Assessment of Pediatric Cancers in India

Domain	Assessment	Solution
Efficiency (maximizing available resources)	India has 26 regional cancer centers and numerous public multi-specialty hospitals with oncology departments.[1] However, there are only 10 pediatric oncology centers in public hospitals[7]	Create space in the existing cancer centers and oncology departments for pediatric cancers
Effectiveness (provide evidence-based healthcare)	ICMR has formulated guidelines for the management of pediatric cancers in India in 2017[8]	Ensure that all oncology centers follow the guidelines The guidelines need to be updated regularly
Equitable care (irrespective of age, gender, financial status, etc.)	80% of healthcare in India is provided by the private sector. This is a paid service, i.e., fee-for-service. Most patients access private healthcare due to the perceived better quality However, with the Universal Health Care Insurance scheme introduced by the Government in 2018, pediatric patients with cancer can access free treatment in private hospitals. Non-governmental organizations like CanKids also sponsor the treatment of poor children with cancer	Ensure that the packages in government schemes are realistic about the cost of treating pediatric cancers Encourage charitable organizations and hospitals to treat children with cancer free of cost by providing them incentives Hospitals should systematically document and share real costs
Safety (avoiding harm)	Pediatric cancer treatment is provided by surgeons, adult medical oncologists, radiation oncologists without formal training in pediatric oncology. This compromises the care as adult protocols are followed, doses are compromised, and toxicities are not managed adequately	Increased pediatric oncology workforce is required. The pediatric oncology fellowship was started a decade ago and 10 doctors graduate every year. This number needs to increase. A dedicated pediatric oncology nursing workforce must be created Safety and quality improvement standards and measures must be routinely integrated into public hospitals
Patient-centered (providing care centered to the patients' needs)	Pediatric cancers are not a priority in India. The true burden of the disease and access to care in India has not been mapped	The patients' and parents' voices and opinions need to be considered It must be ensured that children with cancer have access to care close to home
Timely (reduce the wait time)	Unfortunately, there is a significant delay in referral to cancer centers due to delayed diagnosis, alternative medicine, and financial constraints	Access to treatment closer to the home must be provided. General practitioners must be educated to diagnose and refer cases faster. The public must be educated that alternative medicine does not cure pediatric cancer We can work with alternative medicine practitioners where feasible to manage the symptoms together

ICMR: The Indian Council of Medical Research

Health Quality Domain Assessment of Pediatric Cancers in India

In recent years there has been rapid progress in India in improving its health indicators. As this is evident from its improvements in the infant mortality rate from 50 to 29 per 1000 live births and the under-5 mortality rate from 64 to 36 per 1000 live births between 2008 and 2018.[15] This decline in mortality rate has been achieved through universal vaccination, better perinatal services, and strengthening of primary health care for the management of pneumonia and diarrhea. In the above context, it becomes imperative for the government of India to focus on pediatric cancers as it strides toward the control of infectious diseases and malnutrition.

Thirteen percent of the annual deaths worldwide are cancer-related and 70% of these are in the low- and middle-income countries. Worldwide, the annual number of new cases of childhood cancer exceeds 200,000 and more than 80% of these are from the developing world.[16] Seven out of 10 children with cancer in the resource-rich countries are cured, with a five-year survival for certain cancers, for example, Hodgkin's disease and retinoblastoma, now 95%.[17]

Cancer is generally regarded as a disease of adults. Most populations in the world show incidence of childhood cancer from 75 to 150 per million children per year.[18] However, India reported age of the standardized incidence rate from 38 to 124 per million children per year [Table 1]. Chennai is reported to have the highest incidence and rural Ahmedabad being the lowest of all. This strongly suggests that either there is truly a lesser incidence of childhood cancer in some areas of India, or it is more likely that there is under ascertainment of cases. In urban areas like Bangalore, Bhopal, Chennai, Delhi, Mumbai etc., the reported incidence is generally higher than from rural areas (Barshi and Ahmedabad district) and more comparable with the average world incidence. Again, one can speculate that this can wholly or partly because of under ascertainment of cases and registration in rural areas, but this remains to be confirmed. Further more research is required to investigate if there are factors associated with urban living like overcrowding, air pollution, and so on, which contribute to a relatively higher incidence of childhood cancers in such areas.[16]

Childhood cancer show overall male predominance and the male to female ratio is around 1.2:1 in the most resource-rich countries.[19] In contrast to this, some cancers like retinoblastoma, Wilms' tumor, osteosarcoma, and germ cell tumor actually show a slight female preponderance. In India the reported incidence of childhood cancer in males (39-150 per million children per year) is higher than in females (23-97 per million children per year) in all PBCRs except in North East India [Table 1], and this gives a male to female ratio [Table 2] that is much higher than what is seen in the developed world. One possible explanation for seeking healthcare including treatment of cancer might be gender bias.[20] but one has to also consider other possibilities.

Table 1: Average Annual Number (AAN) of cases of cancer[*] and cancer incidence rates standardized for world population (ASR) in children 0 to 14 years of age[†]

Population based cancer registry[§]	Male			Female			Total		
	AAN[**]	% of all cancer	ASR[††]	AAN	% of all cancer	ASR	AAN	% of all cancer	ASR
Ahmedabad[§] (Rural)	15	3.8	51	5	1.9	23	20	3.1	38
Bangalore (Urban)	69	3.5	87	50	2.1	69	119	2.8	78
Barshi (Rural)	6	5.6	69	4	3.7	53	10	4.6	62
Bhopal (Urban)	16	3.1	58	13	2.8	55	29	2.9	57
Chennai (Urban)	78	3.9	150	47	2.2	97	125	3.0	124
Delhi (Urban)	335	6.5	146	152	3.1	76	487	4.8	113
Mumbai (Urban)	173	3.9	105	117	2.6	79	290	3.2	93
North East[‖]	25	1.2	39	34	2.1	51	59	1.6	45

Table 2: Male to female ratio of major childhood cancer types in each population based cancer registry[*]

Cancer type (ICD 10 Code)	Ahmedabad	Bangalore	Barshi	Bhopal	Chennai	Delhi	Mumbai	North East
Leukemia	0.95	1.20	1.86	0.69	1.55	2.26	1.21	1.09
Lymphoid leukemia (C91)	0.70	1.51	1.32	0.81	1.64	2.60	1.26	1.32
Myeloid leukemia (C92-94)	-[†]	0.77	-	0.29	0.92	1.79	1.54	0.46
Leukemia unspecified (C95)	-	0.32	2.99	0.62	1.82	1.44	0.82	1.41
Lymphoma	-	4.29	1.56	11.26	3.25	4.93	2.19	0.75
Hodgkin's disease (C81)	-	3.84	3.57	-	3.71	11.85	3.11	0.00
Non Hodgkin's lymphoma (C82-85, C96)	-	4.81	0.00	7.78	2.81	3.11	1.74	0.98
Brain, nervous system (C70-72)	-	1.66	2.09	0.31	1.74	1.37	1.65	0.00
Adrenal gland (C74)	-	0.27	-	-	0.81	1.81	1.23	0.00
Eye (C69)	-	0.60	0.90	0.92	1.10	1.90	0.95	1.17
Kidney (C64)	-	1.21	0.00	2.05	1.31	1.31	1.38	1.13
Liver (C22)	-	0.15	-	0.00	0.20	3.04	2.02	-
Bone (C40-41)	-	1.39	1.50	1.10	1.34	1.52	1.23	0.66
Connective and soft tissue (C47, C49)	-	0.83	-	0.82	0.91	1.53	0.82	1.62
Gonadal (C56, C62)	-	0.00	-	0.31	1.16	0.32	0.89	0.88
Other specified and unspecified	1.63	0.83	0.55	5.91	1.12	1.42	0.92	0.31
All Sites	2.24	1.26	1.29	1.07	1.55	1.92	1.34	0.75

The most common childhood cancer in India is Leukemia, proportion varying between 25 and 40%. Of all leukemias reported, 60-85% are acute lymphoblastic leukemia (ALL). T-Cell ALL predominates in economically disadvantaged areas. ALL which peaks in between the age of 2 and 5 years, increases with urbanization, industrialization, and increasing affluence. In India particularly in males, lymphomas often exceed CNS tumors. In India not only is the proportion of lymphomas higher, but Hodgkin's lymphoma (HD) exceeds non-Hodgkin's lymphoma (NHL), whereas in the developed world opposite pattern is seen. There is not very difference in the incidence of HD in females and of NHL in both sexes when compared to the incidence in the developed world. The pathobiology of these cancers is also different. The most common Hodgkin's disease subtype is the mixed cellularity type and it is responsible for the incidence peak at a younger age, as seen in India. The second most common solid tumor in childhood after CNS tumors, is Neuroblastoma but it is less frequently reported in India. Retinoblastoma has an incidence rate of 3 to 5 per million children, per year. Of all childhood cancers in most developed countries, it accounts for 2.5 to 4%.[16]

The reported incidence of childhood cancer has increased over the last 25 years in India, but the increase is much larger in females (44-76% increase) than males (12-27% increase). For leukemias, this striking pattern of sex difference is also seen where there is even higher increase in female children. Whereas CNS tumors shows completely different pattern, of 55-120% increase seen in both sexes. The least increase in incidence is seen in Lymphomas, particularly declined in incidence in female children in Chennai.[21] The disproportionately higher increase in incidence of childhood cancer in females could reflect a shift in the attitude of society toward the female child. Several conclusions can be drawn from these observations but it requires further investigations.

CHAPTER II

ETIOLOGY OF PEDIATRIC CANCERS

The etiology behind childhood cancer have been studied for several decades now. There are few or no strong external risk factors apart from high-dose radiation and prior chemotherapy. Whereas birth weight, parental age, and congenital anomalies are listed under inherent risk factors associated with most types of pediatric cancer. Rarely, a small proportion of cancers are known to be seen in highly-penetrant syndromes. Recently through genome wide association, genetic variation has come into focus as the etiology. These common variations implicated surprisingly in childhood cancers explains a larger proportion of childhood cancers than adult. Through rare variation and non-Mendelian inheritance, maternal genetic effects or de novo germline mutations, may also contribute to risk of development of childhood cancer but further examination is required.

1. ENVIRONMENTAL FACTORS

Environmental exposures that contribute to cancer etiology among children include most of the same exposures known to cause cancer in adults, such as radiation, certain medications, and some industrial and agricultural chemicals. Some childhood exposures such as secondhand cigarette smoke may contribute to cancers that develop many years after childhood. There are also factors suspected of playing a role in childhood cancer but for which the evidence is inconsistent or speculative; for example, electromagnetic fields. For some exposures, such as radiation and pesticides, data suggest that children may be more susceptible to the carcinogenic effects than similarly exposed adults. There are also suggestions of possible interactions between environmental carcinogens and genetic susceptibility.[22]

a. High dose ionizing radiation and prior chemotherapy

The most well-established cause of childhood cancer is radiation. High-dose radiation exposure, such as that experienced by atomic bomb survivors and children receiving radiation therapy for cancer, has caused increases in acute leukemia, chronic mye- logenous leukemia, osteosarcoma, thyroid cancer, breast cancer, and soft tissue sar- coma.[23] Bone sarcomas were also elevated in children treated with radiation and chemotherapy[24].

TABLE 1: SELECTED ENVIRONMENTAL EXPOSURES AND ASSOCIATEDCANCERS AMONG CHILDREN.

EXPOSURE	CANCER
Radiation	Leukemia, thyroid, brain, breast, skin melanoma,a soft tissue sarcoma osteosarcoma
Electromagnetic fields	Leukemia, brain, lymphoma, soft tissue sarcoma
Diethylstilbestrol	Vagina
Phenytoin	Neuroblastoma, soft tissue sarcoma
Alkylating agents	Leukemia, osteosarcoma
Chloramphenicol	Leukemia
Immunosuppressive therapy	Non-Hodgkin's lymphoma, Hodgkin's disease, skin, soft tissue sarcoma
Tobacco	Oral cancer, leukemia, rhabdomyosarcoma, lymphoma, lung cancer
Pesticides	Leukemia, brain cancer, neuroblastoma, Ewing's sarcoma, Wilms' tumor, lymphoma
Epstein-Barr virus	Burkitts' lymphoma

a. Electromagnetic Fields

The EMF generated by power lines, electrical appliances, and large electrical machinery has controversial role in the development of cancer. The consistent exposure to EMF have been found to have increased risk for all leukemia, acute myeloid leukemia, and brain cancer, but the workers usually were also exposed to other potential carcinogens, such as solvents, leaving the role of EMF unclear.[25] Studies of residential EMF exposure have shown associations with leukemia and brain cancer among children, but not among adults.[26] The most puzzling aspect is that the strong association between EMF and childhood leukemia, appeared when EMF was indirectly estimated by evaluating wiring code configurations and appeared weaker when EMF was directly measured.

c. Parental diet caffeine, alcohol use, and vitamin use

Maternal caffeine consumption is associated with caffeine-related risk of childhood leukaemia, including acute lymphocytic (lymphoblastic) leukaemia (ALL), which is the most common cause of death from cancer in children.[27]

Heavy maternal drinking results in fetal alcohol syndrome. As alcohol is known to cross the placenta, it causes deformities and impairments. It is not known if transplacental exposure to alcohol also increases risk of childhood cancer or subsequent cancers in adulthood.[28]

Excessive intake of prenatal vitamin by pregnant mothers was associated with a decreased risk of ALL in offspring.[29]

d. Medication

With the discovery of vaginal adenocarcinoma in 1971 among the daughters of women who took the hormone diethylstilbestrol (DES) during pregnancy to avoid miscarriages, transplacental carcinogenesis was also put in place. It was detected in girls as young as 7 years old, peak between 15 and 22 years of age.[30] Antiepileptic drug, phenytoin was suspected of being a transplacental carcinogen. There were reports of neuroblastoma[31] and soft tissue sarcoma[32] in children exposed in utero to phenytoin.

Also women who used antinausea medications (e.g., Bendectin) during pregnancy, their children reported excess brain tumors, neuroblastomas, leukemia, and retinoblastomas.[33]

Mothers who were exposed to penthrane (methoxyflurane) anesthesia during delivery reported excess Wilms‘ tumor in children.[34]

Parental use of illegal drugs like, Marijuana was associated with rhabdomyosarcoma,[35] leukemia,[36] and brain tumors. Cocaine use was also associated with rhabdomyosarcoma.[37]

e. Paternal and maternal smoking

The parental cigarette smoking have reported increased risk of leukemia and lymphoma, it gets doubled if more than one parent smoked. Rhabdomyosarcoma was associated with paternal but not maternal smoking in one study.[38]

f. Pesticide

Several studies have reported association of pesticides with cancer in adults. Children gets exposed to pesticides from use in homes, gardens, and yards, through the diet, and through contaminated drinking water. Hence, children of farmworkers are often heavily exposed while accompanying their parents to the fields, while in housing contaminated by direct pesticide spray or drift from nearby fields, and through their own farm. The association of neuroblastoma and childhood leukemia with pre and postnatal exposure to termiticide chlordane was reported.[39] In children cases of organophosphate insecticide exposure were linked to aplastic anemia and acute leukemia were reported.[40] Further studies regarding the possible carcinogenic effects, particularly in children is needed.

g. Industrial chemicals and Physical Agents

Children developed mesothelioma decades later who were exposed to the carcinogen asbestos. The asbestos was carried home on their fathers' work clothes or by playing near open pits at an asbestos mine.[41] The roles of other environmental or parental occupational exposures in the development of childhood cancer are unclear. More comprehensive and sensitive methods of assessing exposures by expert industrial hygienists are needed.

h. Air and Drinking water

The fluoridation of municipal drinking water supplies have been evaluated thoroughly many times for the possible carcinogenic effects. On reviewing 36 years of cancer mortality data and 15 years of cancer incidence data, motor vehicle exhaust may also increase the risk of childhood leukemia.[42]

i. Exposure to infections

Generally infectious agents such as viruses have been linked to few types of cancer, but there existed very little evidence. However, it is rare of viral or bacterial induced cancer in children, an exception would be Burkitt's lymphoma, which in Africa is related to infection with Epstein Barr virus.[43]

2. INTRINSIC RISK FACTORS

a. Size for gestational age & optimal birth weight

The accelerated fetal growth is associated with an increased risk of childhood ALL. In children whose birth weight was <4000 g showed association with childhood ALL. Whereas in children with birth weight of >4,000 g, risk of ALL appeared to be little influenced by weight for gestational age.[44]

b. Advanced parental age

Advanced parental age has also showed associated with most childhood cancers. Several research studies were conducted which concluded that significant positive linear trends in leukemia, lymphoma, brain tumor, neuroblastoma, Wilm's tumor, bone tumors, and soft tissue sarcomas with 6-15% increased risk per five years of maternal age.[45]

c. Structural birth defects

Consistently there has been association between structural birth defects and increased risk of childhood cancers. But due to the rarity of both individual birth defects and individual childhood cancers more specific associations have not been reported to date.[46]

d. Genetic risk factors

The known cause of minority of childhood cancers may be the inherited syndromes, caused by high-penetrance germline DNA mutations, chromosomal aneuploidy, or epigenetic disorders.[47] Although 5-10% of syndromes has rarely been precisely quantified for common childhood cancers. For especially rare cancers, such as pediatric adrenocortical carcinoma, the proportion can be much higher.[48]

CHAPTER III

PATHOPHYSIOLOGY OF PEDIATRIC CANCERS

Our understanding of how cancers begin and spread has undergone a significant change over the last half century. Historically, theories invoked to explain the cause of cancer included infectious diseases and nutritional deficiencies. While the development of some cancers can result from infections, we now appreciate that cancers occur as the result of DNA mutations in normal cells. At present, in the modern oncology the damage of the genetic apparatus of the cell is the primary cause of cancer, and the pathogenesis of cancer is seen as a process of transformation of a normal cell into a tumor cell, as evidenced by deep fundamental research of the pathogenesis of cancer, which is held exclusively at the cellular, molecular, and genetic levels of the organism.[49]

In general, cancer cells are distinguished from normal cells by two fundamental properties.

- First, cancers possess abnormalities in the regulation of cell division and survival. Most cells in the human body are not actively dividing at any given moment. Entry into cell cycle is tightly controlled in normal cells. Many cancers, however, have alterations in one or more proteins that regulate mitotic activity. Normal cells also will undergo apoptosis – programmed cell death – because of a variety of conditions including extensive damage to the genome. Cancer cells, however, frequently have alterations in the genes that control apoptosis and, therefore, survive in conditions that would normally be lethal.

- The second characteristic of cancer cells that distinguishes them from normal cells is the ability to metastasize. Metastasis refers to the cancer cells acquired ability to break away from neighboring cells, traverse tissue boundaries, enter and travel through lymphatics and blood vessels, and then grow in foreign tissue environments. It is important to appreciate that cancer is not one disease, but a category of many, which share abnormal cell features.

The shared biologic characteristics of cancerous cells can be classified by their required cellular properties defined as follows:

1. Ability for a cancer to generate mitogenic signals – this is the ability to initiate signal transduction pathways leading to mitosis.

1. Resist exogenous growth-inhibitory signals.

3. Genetic instability- refers to a set of events causing unscheduled alteration within the genome. These changes can be broadly divided into: a) Chromosomal level (i.e. chromosomal gains, loss, translocations, duplications etc.) b) At the nucleotide level (i.e. mutations in DNA repair pathway, mismatch repair pathway defects etc.).

4. Evade apoptosis and acquire unregulated proliferation (immortalized cells).

5. Angiogenesis (growth and proliferation of blood vessels)– required for nutritional support, waste removal and oxygenation to the cancer.

6. Tissue invasion and metastasis through blood or lymphatics.

Tumor refers to “swelling” which may produce a mass. The cause of the mass may be benign or malignant. It is a generic term that may refer to a reactive inflammatory process, an infectious process, benign tissue mass or malignant growth of tissue. It is used interchangeably with neoplasm in the setting of an abnormal tissue growth (either benign or malignant).

Neoplasms are derived from a single clone of cells which grow in an uncoordinated manner. The term neoplasm refers to a clonal growth which can be either benign (non- invasive) or malignant (invasive/cancer). Neoplastic cells must undergo several genetic alterations to overcome the regulated cell growth maintained by normal cells.

- Benign neoplasms are localized expansile masses composed of cells with unregulated cell growth that, with rare exceptions, do not invade tissues and do not metastasize. They often are surrounded by a fibrous capsule and usually easy to surgically resect.

- Malignant neoplasms are masses of unregulated cell growth which are locally invasive and can metastasize. Due to their invasive, irregular border they can be difficult to surgically resect.

The word "cancer" is derived from the Latin word for crab or "karkinos" because of the observed finger-like invasion. Pathologic examination is performed after a biopsy or surgical removal is performed. The evaluation of the cells allows the pathologist to determine whether a neoplasm is benign or malignant. Multiple features must be evaluated by the pathologist to distinguish a benign neoplasm from a malignant neoplasm. When a neoplasm is determined malignant, the neoplastic borders are assessed for evidence of infiltration and into normal tissue.

A well differentiated malignancy has features like the tissue of origin. However, poorly differentiated malignancies do not appear anything like components of the precursor organ, thereby making determination of tumor origin more challenging. A low grade (grade 1) indicates a well-differentiated malignancy, whereas a high grade (grade 3) indicates a poorly differentiated malignancy. The grade of the malignancy (differentiation) is a key component of a pathologic assessment.

Regardless of difference in types of cancer histologically and physiologically, there is existence of a common pathophysiological process of malignant tumors or cancer development in the organism. The commonly accepted basis of the pathogenesis of cancer is the damage to the genetic apparatus of cells (such as mutation, disturbance of gene expression, activation of tumor promoter gene, inactivation of tumor suppressor genes, etc.). It is believed that damage to the genetic apparatus of the cell along with inactivation of anti-tumor genes takes place and is essential for the development of malignant tumors. But it should be noted that the inactivation of tumor suppressor gene is one of the natural physiological reactions of the organism, and when this reaction becomes pathophysiological condition of an organism it results in cancer development.

At the cellular level, the development of cancer is viewed as a multi-step process involving mutation and selection for cells with progressively increasing capacity for proliferation, survival, invasion, and metastasis.

First step: Mutation and tumor initiation

- Genetic alteration leads to mutation in a single cell which results into abnormal proliferation of that cell known as tumor cell.

Second step: Cell proliferation and Tumor progression

- Tumor progression continues as additional mutations occur within cells of the tumor population.
- The mutated cells have some selective advantage over normal cell as such cells shows rapid growth and division. The descendants of a cell bearing such additional mutation will consequently become dominant within the tumor population.

Third step: Clonal selection andmalignancy

- Cell proliferation of tumor then leads to new clone of tumor cells with increased growth rate or other properties (such as survival, invasion, or metastasis) that confer a selective advantage. The process is called clonal selection.
- Clonal selection continues throughout tumor development, so tumors continuously become more rapid-growing and increasingly malignant.
- **For example:** In colon cancer, the earliest stage in tumor development is increased proliferation of colon epithelial cells. A clonal selection occurs in which, a single cell within these proliferative cell population give rise to a small benign neoplasm.

Further rounds of clonal selection led to the growth of benign neoplasm with increase in size and proliferative potential resulting in malignant carcinoma. The cancer cells then continue to proliferate and spread through the connective tissues of the colon wall. Eventually the cancer cells penetrate the wall of the colon and invade other abdominal organs, such as the bladder or small intestine. In addition, the cancer cells invade blood and lymphatic vessels, allowing them to metastasize throughout the body.

Fourth step: Metastasis

- **Metastasis** is a complex process in which cancer cells break away from the primary tumor and circulate through the bloodstream or lymphatic system to other sites in the body.
- At new sites, the cells continue to multiply and eventually form additional tumors comprised of cells that reflect the tissue of origin.
- The ability of tumors, such as pancreatic cancer and uveal (iris, ciliary body, or choroid of eye) cancers, to metastasize contributes greatly to their lethality.
- Many fundamental questions remain about the clonal structures of metastatic tumors, phylogenetic relationships among metastases, the scale of ongoing parallel evolution in metastatic and primary sites, how the tumor disseminates, and the role that the tumor micro-environment plays in the determination of the metastatic site.

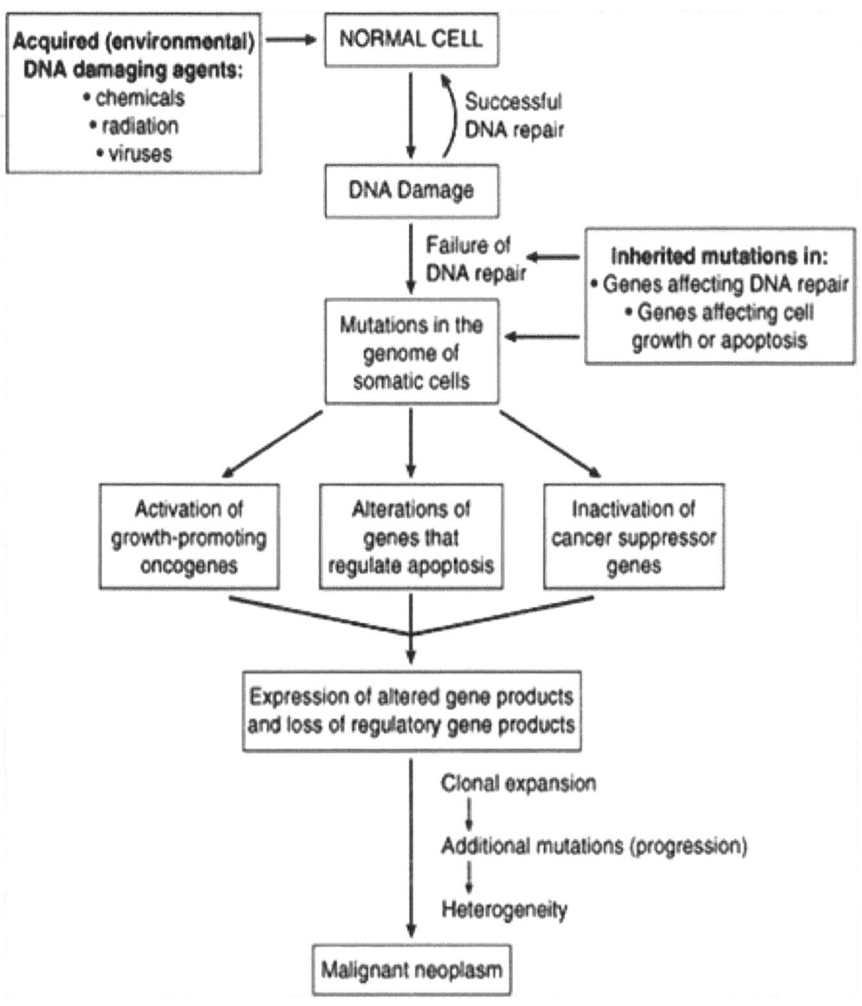

Fig. No.1 Pathophysiology of pediatric cancers

CHAPTER IV

CLASSIFICATION OF PEDIATRIC CANCERS

<u>INTERNATIONAL CLASSIFICATION OF CHILDHOOD CANCER (1996)</u>

1. Leukemia

    a. Lymphoid Leukemia Excluding ALL

    a. Acute Leukemia Excluding AML

    c. Chronic Myeloid Leukemia

    d. Other Specified Leukemias

    e. Unspecified Leukemias

2. Lymphomas and Reticuloendothelial Neoplasms

    a. Hodgkin's disease

    b. Non-Hodgkin's lymphomas

    c. Burkitt's lymphoma

    d. Miscellaneous Lymphoreticular neoplasms

    e. Unspecified lymphomas

3. CNS and Miscellaneous Intracranial and Intraspinal Neoplasms

    a. Ependymoma

    b. Astrocytoma

   c. Primitive neurectodermal tumors
   d. Other gliomas
   e. Miscellaneous intracranial and intraspinal neoplasms
   f. Unspecified intracranial and intraspinal neoplasms
4. Sympathetic Nervous System Tumors
   a. Neuroblastoma and ganglioneuroblastoma
   b. Other sympathetic nervous system tumors
5. Retinoblastoma
6. Renal Tumors
   a. Wilms' tumor, rhabdoid and clear cell sarcoma
   b. Renal carcinoma
   c. Unspecified malignant renal tumors
7. Hepatic Tumors
   a. Hepatoblastoma
   b. Hepatic carcinoma
   c. Unspecified malignant hepatic tumors
8. Malignant Bone Tumors
   a. Osteosarcoma
   b. Chrondosarcoma

    c. Ewing's sarcoma
    d. Other specified malignant bone tumors
    e. Unspecified malignant bone tumors

9. Soft-Tissue Sarcomas
    a. Rhabdomyosarcoma and embryonal sarcoma
    b. Fibrosarcoma, neurofibrosarcoma and other fibromatous neoplasms
    c. Kaposi's sarcoma
    d. Other specified soft tissue sarcomas
    e. Unspecified soft-tissue sarcomas
10. Germ-Cell, Trophoblastic and other gonadal neoplasms
    a. Intracranial and intra spinal germ-cell tumors
    b. Other and unspecified non-gonadal germ-cell tumors
    c. Gonadal germ-cell tumors
    d. Gonadal carcinomas
    e. Other and unspecified malignant gonadal tumors
11. Carcinomas and other Malignant Epithelial Neoplasms
    a. Adrenocortical carcinoma
    b. Thyroid carcinoma
    c. Nasopharyngeal carcinoma

d. Malignant melanoma

e. Skin carcinoma

f. Other and unspecified carcinomas

12. Other and Unspecified Malignant Neoplasms

a. Other specified malignant tumors

b. Other unspecified malignant tumors

WHO CLASSIFICATION OF PEDIATRIC TUMORS

Classification of pediatric leukemias and lymphomas

1. Myeloid neoplasms

a. Myeloproliferative neoplasms

- Chronic myeloid leukemia, BCR::ABL1 positive

b. Myelodysplastic/myeloproliferative neoplasms

- Juvenile myelomonocytic leukemia

c. Myelodysplastic syndromes

- Refractory cytopenia of childhood
- Myelodysplastic syndrome with excess blasts

d. Myeloid neoplasms with germline predisposition

e. Myeloid proliferations associated with Down syndrome

f. Acute myeloid leukemia and related neoplasms

- Acute myeloid leukemia, NOS
- Acute myeloid leukemia with recurrent genetic abnormalities

- AML with t(8;21)(q22;q22); RUNX1::RUNX1T1
- AML with inv(16)(p13.1q22) or t(16;16)(p13.1;q22); CBFB::MYH11
- APL with t(15;17)(q24.1;q21.2); PML::RARA
- AML with KMT2A-rearrangement new
- AML with t (6;9) (p23; q34.1); DEK:: NUP214
- AML with inv(3)(q21q26)/t(3;3)(q21;q26); GATA2, RPN1::MECOM
- AML with ETV6-fusion new
- AML with t(8;16)(p11.2;p13.3); KAT6A::CREBBP new
- AML with t(1;22)(p13.3;q13.1); RBM15::MKL1
- AML with CBFA2T3::GLIS2 (inv(16)(p13q24)) new
- AML with NUP98-fusion new

- AML with t(16;21)(p11;q22); FUS::ERG new
- AML with mutated NPM1
- AML with bZIP mutated CEBPA

2. Mast cell neoplasia

   (a) Mastocytosis

   Lymphoid neoplasms

a. Precursor lymphoid neoplasms

- B-cell lymphoblastic leukemia/lymphomas
- B-LBLL with t(9;22)(q34.1;q11.2); BCR::ABL1
- B-LBLL with t(v;11q23.3); KMT2A-rearranged
- B-LBLL with t(12;21)(p13.2;q22.1); ETV6::RUNX1
- B-LBLL with hypodiploidy, near- haploid
- B-LBLL with hypodiploidy, low
- B-LBLL with hypodiploidy, high
- B-LBLL with t(5;14)(q31.1;q32.1); IGH::IL3
- B-LBLL with t(1;19)(q23;p13.3); TCF3::PBX1
- B-LBLL, BCR::ABL1-like (Philadelphia-like B-ALL)
- B-LBLL with iAMP21
- T-cell and natural killer (NK)-cell lymphoblastic leukemia/lymphoma
- T-lymphoblastic leukemia/lymphoma

- Early T-cell precursor lymphoblastic leukemia
- NK-lymphoblastic leukemia/lymphoma

b. Mature B-cell neoplasms

- Primary mediastinal (thymic) large B-cell lymphoma
- Diffuse large B-cell lymphoma, NOS
- EBV-positive diffuse large B-cell lymphoma, NOS
- Large B-cell lymphoma with IRF4 rearrangement
- Pediatric-type follicular lymphoma

- Pediatric nodal marginal zone lymphoma
- ALK-positive large B-cell lymphoma
- Lymphomatoid granulomatosis
- Plasmablastic lymphoma
- Grey-zone lymphoma
- Burkitt lymphoma- Burkitt-like lymphoma with 11q aberration

c. Mature T/NK-cell neoplasms

- Peripheral T cell lymphoma
- Aggressive NK-cell leukemia
- Mycosis fungoides- Anaplastic large cell lymphoma, ALK-positive
- Hepatosplenic T-cell lymphoma
- Primary cutaneous CD30+ T-cell lymphoproliferative disorders
- Systemic EBV+ T-cell lymphoma of childhood
- Hydroa vacciniforme lymphoproliferative disorder
- Subcutaneous panniculitis-like T-cell lymphoma

d. Hodgkin lymphoma

- Classical Hodgkin lymphoma
- Nodular lymphocyte predominant Hodgkin lymphoma

e. Histiocytic and dendritic cell neoplasms

- Langerhans cell histiocytosis and other histiocytic/dendritic cell neoplasms

f. Immunodeficiency-associated lymphoproliferative disorders

- Primary immunodeficiency associated lymphoproliferative disorders
- Post-transplant lymphoproliferative disorders
- HIV-associated lymphoproliferative disorders

Classification of pediatric soft-tissue and bone tumors
Soft-Tissue Tumors

1. Adipocytic tumors

- Lipomatosis
- Lipoblastoma/lipoblastomatosis
- Liposarcoma

2. Fibroblastic and myofibroblastic tumors

- Fasciitis
- Fibrodysplasia ossificans progressivaa new
- Fibroma of tendon sheath
- Gardner fibroma
- Fibrous hamartoma of Infancy
- Lipofibromatosis
- Inclusion body infantile digital fibromatosis
- Juvenile hyaline fibromatois (Hyaline fibromatosis syndrome)
- Fibromatosis colli
- Calcifying aponeurotic fibroma
- Sinonasal angiofibroma
- Plantar/palmar fibromatoses
- Desmoid fibromatosis- EWSR1::SMAD3 positive fibroblastic tumor
- Infantile fibrosarcoma- Pediatric NTRK-rearranged spindle cell neoplasm (provisional entity)
- Dermatofibrosarcoma protuberans/Giant cell fibroblastoma
- Low-grade fibromyxoid sarcoma/Sclerosing epithelioid
- Low-grade myofibroblastic sarcoma
- Inflammatory myofibroblastic tumor

3. So-called fibrohistiocytic tumors

- Fibrous histiocytoma
- Plexiform fibrohistiocytic tumor

- Tenosynovial giant cell tumor

4. Vascular tumors

- Capillary malformations
- Venous malformations (Venous hemangioma)
- Arteriovenous malformations (Arteriovenous malformation/ hemangioma)
- Intramuscular vascular anomalies (Intramuscular hemangioma)
- Lymphatic anomalies (Lymphangioma and lymphangiomatosis)
- Congenital hemangioma
- Infantile hemangioma
- Hemangioma of placenta
- Pyogenic granuloma
- Epithelioid Hemangioma
- Tufted angioma and kaposiform hemangioendothelioma
- Papillary intralymphatic angioendothelioma (PILA) and retiform - hemangioendothelioma
- Pseudomyogenic hemangiendothelioma
- Kaposi sarcoma
- Epithelioid hemangioendothelioma
- Angiosarcoma

5. Pericytic (perivascular) tumors

- Myofibroma and myopericytoma
- Glomus tumor and glomuvenous malformation

6. Smooth muscle tumors

- EBV-associated smooth muscle tumor

7. Skeletal muscle tumors

- Rhabdomyoma

- Rhabdomyosarcoma family
- Ectomesenchymoma

8. Gastrointestinal stromal tumor

    - Pediatric gastrointestinal stromal tumor (GIST)

9. Peripheral nerve sheath tumors

    - Schwannoma
    - Neurofibroma
    - Perineurioma
    - Hybrid nerve sheath tumor
    - Granular cell tumor
    - Solitary circumscribed neuroma
    - Ectopic meningioma and meningothelial hamartoma
    - Benign triton tumor/neuromuscular choristoma
    - Malignant peripheral nerve sheath tumor

10. Tumors of uncertain differentiation

    - Tumors of uncertain differentiation
    - Intramuscular/Juxta-articular myxoma
    - Superficial angiomyxoma
    - Deep angiomyxoma
    - Angiomatoid fibrous histiocytoma
    - Clear cell sarcoma of soft tissue
    - Alveolar soft part sarcoma
    - Extrarenal rhabdoid tumor
    - PEComa
    - Synovial sarcoma
    - Epithelioid sarcoma
    - Myoepithelial tumors of soft tissue
    - Phosphaturic mesenchymal tumor
    - Desmoplastic small round cell tumor
    - Undifferentiated sarcomas (non-small cell round cells)

11. Undifferentiated small round cell sarcomas of bone and soft tissue

- Undifferentiated small round cell sarcomas of bone and soft tissue
- Ewing sarcoma
- Round cell sarcoma with EWSR1–non-ETS fusions
- CIC-rearranged sarcomas
- Sarcoma with BCOR genetic alterations

Bone Tumors

1. Osteogenic tumors

- Subungual exostosis
- Bizarre parosteal osteochondromatous proliferation
- Osteoblastoma
- Osteoid osteoma
- Chondromesenchymal hamartoma of chest wall
- Osteosarcoma

2. Chondrogenic tumors

- Chondroblastoma
- Osteochondroma
- Chondromyxoid fibroma
- Enchondroma and enchondromatosis
- Chondrosarcoma
- Mesenchymal chondrosarcoma

3. Other tumors

- Vascular tumors of bone
- Aneurysmal bone cyst (ABC)
- Giant cell tumor of bone (GCTB)
- Non-ossifying fibroma (NOF)
- Notochordal tumors
- Simple bone cyst

- Adamantinoma
- Osteofibrous dysplasia (OFD)
- Fibrous dysplasia

Classification of pediatric solid tumors

1. Peripheral neuroblastic tumors

   - Ganglioneuroma
   - Ganglioneuroblastoma, intermixed
   - Neuroblastoma
   - Ganglioneuroblastoma, nodular (and other composite neuroblastic tumors)

2. Eye tumors

   - Conjunctival Neoplasms
   - Hamartomas
   - Epibulbar choristoma
   - Epibulbar osseous choristoma
   - Phakomatous choristoma
   - Melanocytic Neoplasms
   - Conjunctival junctional, compound, and subepithelial nevi
   - Inflamed juvenile conjunctival nevus

3. Uveal Neoplasms

   - Hamartomas
   - Diffuse choroidal neurofibroma and ganglioneuroma
   - Lisch nodule (iris hamartoma)

4. Retinal and neuroepithelial tumors

   - Retinocytoma
   - Retinoblastoma
   - Medulloepithelioma

5. Optic nerve tumors

   - Pilocytic astrocytoma and other gliomas of the optic nerve

6. Germ cell tumors

- Non-invasive germ cell neoplasia
- Intratubular germ cell neoplasia (Male gonadal)
- Gonadoblastoma
- Germinoma family
- Germinoma/Dysgerminoma/Seminoma (new as a unifying entity)
- Nongerminomatous germ cell tumors
- Mature cystic teratoma
- Extra-gonadal teratoma
- Monodermal teratomas (Female gonadal)
- Immature teratoma (Female gonadal)
- Prepubertal type testicular teratoma
- Post-pubertal type teratoma
- Embryonal carcinoma
- Yolk sac tumor
- Fetus in fetu
- Choriocarcinoma (nongestational)
- Malignant mixed germ cell tumor

7. Renal and male genital tumors

- Kidney
- Nephroblastic and related tumors
- Pediatric cystic nephroma
- Nephroblastoma
- Molecularly defined renal tumors
- Renal cell carcinoma with MIT translocations
- ALK driven renal cell carcinoma
- Eosinophilic, solid and cystic (ESC) renal cell carcinoma (TSC related)
- SMARCB1-deficient renal medullary carcinoma

- Metanephric tumors
- Metanephric adenoma
- Metanephric adenofibroma
- Metanephric stromal tumor
- Mesenchymal renal tumors
- Ossifiying renal tumor of infancy
- Mesoblastic nephroma

- Clear cell sarcoma of kidney
- Malignant rhabdoid tumor of the kidney
- Anaplastic sarcoma of kidney
- Renal Ewing sarcoma

8. Testis

    - Juvenile granulosa cell tumor of the testis

9. Female genital tumors

    - Ovary
    - Sex cord-stromal tumors
    - Ovarian fibroma
    - Sclerosing stromal tumor
    - Juvenile granulosa cell tumor of the ovary
    - Sex cord tumor with annular tubules
    - Papillary cystadenoma
    - Sertoli-Leydig tumor
    - Gynandroblastoma
    - Other
    - Small cell carcinoma of ovary, hypercalcemic type
    - Lower female genital tumors
    - Epithelial tumors
    - Mullerian papilloma
    - Mesonephric remnants and hyperplasia
    - Condyloma acuminatum

    - Peritoneum
    - Mesothelial tumors
    - Peritoneal inclusion cysts
    - Breast tumors
    - Fibroepithelial tumors
    - Juvenile fibroadenoma
    - Juvenile papillomatosis

10. Digestive system tumors

- Liver
- Epithelial tumors
- Hepatoblastoma
- Fibrolamellar variant of hepatocellular carcinoma
- Pediatric hepatocellular carcinoma new
- Mesenchymal tumors unique to liver
- Mesenchymal hamartoma
- Calcifying nested stromal-epithelial tumor
- Embryonal sarcoma of the liver
- Hepatic congenital hemangioma new
- Hepatic infantile hemangioma new
- Hepatic angiosarcoma
- Pancreas
- Epithelial tumors
- Pancreatoblastoma
- Pancreatic acinar cell carcinoma
- Solid pseudopapillary neoplasm
- Gastrointestinal tract
- Epithelial tumors
- Gastroblastoma
- Appendiceal NETs

11. Endocrine tumors

- Thyroid
- Thyroid epithelial tumors
- Follicular adenoma of the thyroid
- Papillary thyroid carcinoma
- Medullary thyroid carcinoma
- Spindle epithelial tumor with thymus-like elements
- Parathyroid
- Parathyroid endocrine tumors
- Parathyroid adenoma
- Adrenal
- Adrenocortical tumors
- Tumors of the adrenal medulla and extra-adrenal paraganglia
- Sympathetic paraganglioma
- Parasympathetic paraganglioma (H&N paraganglioma)

- Pheochromocytoma
- Composite pheochromocytoma/paraganglioma
- Neuroendocrine neoplasms

12. Head and neck tumors

- Benign
- Squamous cell papilloma of larynx
- White sponge nevus new
- Congenital granular cell epulis
- Central giant cell granuloma
- Odontogenic tumors
- Ossifying fibroma
- Sino-nasal tract myxoma
- Nasal dermoid cyst
- Nasopharyngeal dermoid Nasal chondromesenchymal hamartoma
- Pleomorphic adenoma
- Malignant

- Mucoepidermoid carcinoma
- Acinic cell carcinoma
- Sialoblastoma
- Nasopharyngeal carcinoma NUT carcinoma
- Melanotic neuroectodermal tumor of infancy

13. Thoracic tumors

- Lung
- Fetal lung interstitial tumor new
- Congenital peribronchial myofibroblastic tumor
- Pleuropulmonary blastoma
- Heart
- Cardiac rhabdomyoma

14. Skin tumors

- Hamartomas
- Epithelial Neoplasms

- Squamous
- Angiokeratoma
- Epidermal nevi (nevus sebaceus)
- Pilomatricoma
- Melanocytic neoplasms
- Nevi
- Congenital neviJunctional, compound, and dermal nevi
- Blue nevus and cellular blue nevus
- Spitz nevus
- Pigmented spindle cell nevus (Reed nevus)
- Melanoma

Classification of pediatric CNS tumors

1. **Gliomas, glioneuronal, and neuronal tumors**

- Pediatric-type diffuse low-grade gliomas
- Diffuse astrocytoma, MYB or MYBL1-altered
- Angiocentric glioma
- Polymorphous low-grade neuroepithelial tumor of the young
- Diffuse low-grade glioma, MAPK pathway-altered
- Pediatric-type diffuse high-grade gliomas defined by H3 status
- Diffuse midline glioma, H3 K27-altered
- Diffuse hemispheric glioma, H3 G34-mutant
- Diffuse pediatric-type high-grade glioma, H3-wild-type and IDH-wild-type
- Infant-type hemispheric glioma
- Circumscribed astrocytic gliomas
- Pilocytic astrocytoma
- High-grade astrocytoma with piloid features
- Pleomorphic xanthoastrocytoma
- Subependymal giant cell astrocytoma
- Astroblastoma, MN1-altered
- Glioneuronal and neuronal tumors
- Ganglioglioma
- Desmoplastic infantile ganglioglioma/Desmoplastic infantile astrocytoma
- Dysembryoplastic neuroepithelial tumor

- Diffuse glioneuronal tumor with oligodendroglioma-like features and nuclear clusters (DGONC)
- Diffuse leptomeningeal glioneuronal tumor
- Multinodular and vacuolating neuronal tumor
- Ependymal tumors
- Supratentorial ependymoma
- Supratentorial ependymoma, ZFTA fusion–positive
- Supratentorial ependymoma, YAP1 fusion–positive
- Posterior fossa ependymoma

- Posterior fossa ependymoma, Group PFA
- Posterior fossa ependymoma, Group PFB
- Spinal ependymoma, MYCN-amplified
- Myxopapillary ependymoma

2. Choroid plexus tumors

    - Choroid plexus papilloma
    - Atypical choroid plexus papilloma
    - Choroid plexus carcinoma

3. CNS embryonal tumors

    - Medulloblastomas, molecularly defined
    - Medulloblastoma, WNT-activated
    - Medulloblastoma, SHH-activated & TP53-wild-type
    - Medulloblastoma, SHH-activated & TP53-mutant
    - Medulloblastoma, non-WNT/non-SHH
    - Medulloblastoma, histologically defined
    - Medulloblastoma, histologically defined
    - Other CNS embryonal tumors
    - Atypical teratoid/rhabdoid tumor
    - Cribriform neuroepithelial tumor
    - Embryonal tumor with multilayered rosettes
    - CNS neuroblastoma, FOXR2-activated
    - CNS tumor with BCOR internal tandem duplication
    - CNS embryonal tumor NEC/NOS

4. Pineal region tumors

    - Pineoblastoma

5. Melanocytic tumors

    - Meningeal melanocytosis and melanomatosis

6. Tumors of the sellar region

    - Pituitary endocrine tumors
    - Pituitary adenoma/PitNET
    - Pituitary blastoma
    - Craniopharyngiomas
    - Adamantinomatous craniopharyngioma

CHAPTER V

TYPE OF PEDIATRIC CANCERS

A. LUKEMIA

- INTRODUCTION
- ETIOLOGY
- PATHOPHYSIOLOGY
- CLASSIFICATION
- ORAL MANIFESTATIONS
- DENTAL MANAGEMENT
- DENTAL COMPLICATIONS

• INTRODUCTION

One of the most common cancer in children is Leukemia. There is steady increase in the incidence which strongly indicates the origins of childhood leukemia are influenced not only by genetics. Studies support those environmental chemical exposures and altered patterns of infection during early development may play an important role.[52] Most leukemia diagnoses in children are sporadic.

There are 3 main subtypes of leukemia: acute lymphoblastic leukemia (ALL), acute myelogenous leukemia (AML), and chronic myelogenous leukemia (CML). ALL is the most common subtype, accounting for approximately 80% of cases. CML is the least common. There are many subgroups within ALL and AML. It is important to know that patients are affected and treated differently for each type of leukemia. One thing in common amongst these 4 types of leukemia is that they begin in a cell in the bone marrow. The cell undergoes a change and becomes a type of leukemia cell. These subgroups have variable biological features, prognoses, and treatment regimens. Children generally present with symptoms related to cytopenias or leukemic infiltration of the bone marrow. Other organs, such as the spleen, liver, testes, and central nervous system (CNS), can also be involved. With modern, risk-adapted therapy, most children are cured of their disease. Despite these successes, relapse continues to be a problem.

However, we have entered an exciting time of targeted and immunologic therapy that is revolutionizing the treatment of these challenging patients.

- **ETIOLOGY** (Table no.2)

1. Genetics

In the etiology of leukemia, undoubtedly genetics plays a major role. For most leukemia cases there are no obvious known predisposing factors, but the increased incidence of leukemia may be associated with some genetic and acquired germline mutations and clonal chromosomal abnormalities. The germline mutations that can cause leukemia prone changes have been identified increasingly using genome-wide association studies. Patients with DNA repair disorders and constitutional chromosomal anomalies can be susceptible to the development of leukemia. In the absence of extramedullary phenotypes, some inherited mutations have the potential to enhance the risk of developing leukemia. Some families have an increased incidence of leukemia with no known inherited mutations.[53] The major inherited and genetic disorders resulting in a predisposition to acute leukemia are summarized in Table below.

The identified genes that can be inherited in an autosomal dominant fashion and potentially result in the development of leukemia include CEPBA, RUNX1 and GATA2.

- CEBPA gene, located at chromosome19q13.1, encodes granulocytic differentiation factor C/EBPa, a member of the bZIP family of proteins.

- RUNX1 gene is located at 21q22.12 and is a transcription factor involved in hemopoiesis.

- GATA2 gene is located at 3q21.3 and is involved in preserving the integrity of hematopoietic stem cells and regulating phagocytosis.[54]

Predisposing Disorder	Gene	Inheritance	Type of Leukemia
CEBPA	*CEBPA*	AD	MDS/AML
Monosomy 7	*7p/q*	AD	MDS/AML/ALL
Familial platelet disorder/AML	*RUNX1*	AD	MDS/AML/T-cell ALL
MonoMAC Syndrome	*GATA2*	AD	MDS/AML
Familial AML with mutated DDX41	*DDX41*	AD	MDS/AML/CMML
Thrombocytopenia 2	*ANKRD26*	AD	MDS/AML
Thrombocytopenia 5	*ETV6*	AD	MDS/AM/CMML, B-cell ALL
Familial MDS/AML with mutated GATA2	*GATA2*	AD	MDS/AML/CMML
Li-Fraumeni syndrome	*TP53*	AD	ALL
Neurofibromatosis type 1	*NF1*	AD	JMML/MDS/AML
Noonan syndrome	*PTPN11*	AD	JMML/MDS/AML
CBL syndrome	*CBL*	AD	JMML
Familial aplastic anemia with mutated SRP72	*SRP72*	AD	MDS/AML
Familial B- cell ALL with mutated PAX5	*PAX5*	AD	ALL
Germline SH2B3	*SH2B3*	AR	ALL
Telomere syndromes (dyskeratosis congenita)	*TERC, TERT, CTC1, DKC1, NHP2, NOP10, RTEL1, TINF2, WRAP53, ACD, PARN*	AD, AR	MDS/AML
Diamond Blackfan anemia	*RPS19, RPL5, RPL11*	Sporadic, AD, AR,	MDS/AML/ALL
Shwachman-Diamond syndrome	*SBDS*	AR	MDS/AML/ALL
Amegakaryocytic thrombocytopenia	*c-MPL*	AR	MDS/AML
Thrombocytopenia with absent radii syndrome	*RBM8A*	AR, Sporadic	ALL/AML
Severe congenital neutropenia	*ELA2, HAX1, G6PC3, WASP*	AD, AR, X-linked	MDS/AML
Fanconi anemia	*FANCA, FANCB, FANCC, BRCA2, FANCD2, FANCE, FANCF, FANCG, FANCI, BRIP1, FANCL, FANCM, PALB2, RAD51C, SLX4*	AR	ALL/AML
Mismatch repair Cancer syndrome	*PMS2, MSH6, MLH1, MSH2*	AR	ALL
Ataxia-telangiectasia	*ATM*	AR	ALL
Nijmegen breakage syndrome	*NBS1*	AR	ALL
Bloom Syndrome	*BLM*	AR	ALL
Werner Syndrome	*WRN (RECQL2)*	AR	MDS/AML
Rothmund-Thomson	*RECQL4*	AR	AML
Wiskott-Aldrich Syndrome	*WASP*	X-linked	ALL
Burton's agammaglobulinemia	*BTK*	X-linked	ALL
Trisomy 21 (Down Syndrome)	*21q*	Sporadic	ALL/AML

AD—autosomal dominant, AR—autosomal recessive, MDS—myelodysplastic syndrome, ALL—acute lymphoblastic leukemia, AML—acute myeloblastic leukemia, JMML—juvenile myelo-monocytic leukemia, CMML—chronic myelomonocytic leukemia.

(Table no.2) : Etiology

2. Environment and Occupations

Many environmental causes for the development of leukemia have been suggested. These mostly involve exposure to cancer-causing agents, including chemicals, infections and radiation during various stages of life.[55-59] Certain exposures, occupations, industrial hazards, and hobbies have been implicated in a higher risk of leukemia.[60] The relation of certain occupations and the occurrence of acute leukemias is not certain and at times controversial.

Industries with Increased Rate of Leukemia
Agriculture/Crop production and related ventures
Forestry
Fishing and Hunting
Construction and related services
Animal slaughtering/poultry processing
Oil refining and petrochemicals
Industries with Decreased Rate of Acute Leukemia
Professional, legal and technical services
Computer systems and related services
Business support, management and administrative services
Public administration

Occupations described to be associated with increased risk for leukemias include, but are not limited to, agricultural and forestry work and crop production[61] with exposure to pesticides and fertilizers,[62] construction,[63] animal slaughtering and poultry work, vocations in the oil/gas industries with exposure to benzene, oil refining and petrochemicals, automobile mechanic works, electrical utility careers, jobs with exposure to magnetic fields, works in the nuclear power industry/exposure to ionizing radiation, furniture manufacturing/repair and nursing and health care positions with exposure to infectious agents/viruses. Other occupations with increased risk of leukemia include hairdressing and hair dying, painting, laundry work, dry-cleaning with exposure to dry-cleaning chemicals, teachers, workers in the shoe and boot manufacturing industry and taxi, bus, truck, and railway drivers and conductors. Occupations with exposure to alkylating agents and formaldehyde, textile workers and manufacturers and semiconductor workers are also found to have a higher risk of leukemia. Increased risk of leukemia due to contact with workers in these industries is suggested.[61-64]

Occupations Associated with Increased Risk of Acute Leukemia
Farmers, foresters, agriculture workers and related occupations
Fishing and related works
Construction, painting, maintenance and related occupations
Carpet, tile and floor installers
Building and ground cleaning, janitorial and maintenance workers
Healthcare workers
Workers exposed to solvents, chemicals and benzene
Electricians/electrical utility workers
Workers exposed to high doses of radiation/nuclear power industry
Automobile mechanics/drivers/rail conductors and pilots
Furniture manufacturers and repair personnel
Laundry workers, dry cleaners
Textile workers and manufacturers
Hairdressers
Teachers
Occupations Associated with Decreased Risk of Acute Leukemia
Attorneys and legal workers
Movers

3. Effects of Radiation

In the development of leukemia, effect of ionizing radiation is seen at various phases of life, including preconception, in utero, and post-natal exposures. The dose of irradiation and the occurrence of leukemia has been reported to show the correlation.[65] Some studies reported an elevated risk for childhood leukemia related to paternal diagnostic X-rays. If two or more X-rays of the lower abdomen were done, an increased risk was found. Hence a correlation between diagnostic X-rays and the development of leukemia is inconsistent, inconclusive, and subject to several variables, including time and reason for the procedure and statistical errors. Inconsistent results regarding exposure to nonionizing radiation and the development of leukemia have been disputed.[66,67]

4. Prior Immunosuppressive and Chemotherapy

An increased risk of leukemia is seen in individuals who have received chemotherapy for the treatment of cancer, with or without radiation. The immunosuppressive therapies and certain chemotherapeutic agents are associated with an increased risk of developing acute leukemias. The chemotherapy agents, such as alkylating agents, platinum derivates and topoisomerase II inhibitors, are shown to be associated with the disease.

The addition of radiation therapy to chemotherapy also increases the risk involved.[68]

5. Parental and Residential Factors

In the pediatrics, paternal hobbies, and occupations, such as work involving contact with gasoline, paint, pigments, solvents, pesticide and plastics, jobs in metal, textile, pharmaceutical industries and professions requiring engine repair, have been investigated for the development of leukemia in children. Direct and indirect effects of chemical agents on children, including via breastfeeding and exposure to contaminated clothing or environment, have been implicated.[69]

- Household exposure to pesticides and insecticides has been found to be associated with a higher risk of leukemia in the pediatric age group.[70]
- The proximity of place of birth to the industrial sites with release of volatile organic compounds has been reported.[71]
- Children born through in vitro fertilization have a higher rate of acute leukemia and Hodgkin's lymphoma.[72]
- Parental alcohol consumption and smoking during prenatal and neonatal periods and childhood have been suggested to contribute to the development of leukemia in their offspring. The risk may be related to the severity, frequency, duration and extent of the exposure.[73]
- Maternal use of marijuana during and after pregnancy has been reported to increase the risk of ALL and AML by 10-fold.[74]

6. Maternal and paternal age

A positive association between maternal and paternal age greater than 35 and 40 years, respectively, and the occurrence of ALL in the offspring was found. Maternal and paternal age exceeding 40 years has been reported to be associated with the development of childhood leukemia.[75]

7. Infections

Infections such as bacterial, viral and fungal agents alone, and in conjunction with genetic mutations, have been implicated in leukemogenesis. Infective agents have been suspected to be associated with the development of cancer in general and acute leukemias.[76] During the first two years of life, exposure to EBV resulting in a positive serological response and the development of Burkitt's lymphoma has been reported.[77] Carcinogenic effects of fungal agents and aflatoxin are well established, but the mechanisms resulting in this phenomenon are not entirely clear. The correlation between exposure to infections, including fungal organisms, and occupations with increased rate of leukemia, such as agricultural work, which potentially exposes the workers to fungal and other agents is not clear and requires future investigation.

- **PATHOPHYSIOLOGY**

Due to the malignant transformation of pluripotent (i.e., can give rise to both myeloid and lymphoid precursors) hematopoietic stem cells, leukemia occurs. Sometimes a more committed stem cell that has a limited self-renewal capacity can also get involved in the process. In case of acute leukemias, these malignant cells are generally immature, poorly differentiated, abnormal leukocytes (blasts) that can either be lymphoblasts or myeloblasts. Further these blasts like cells undergo clonal expansion and proliferation, leading to replacement and interference of the development and the function of normal blood products with malignant cells, leading to clinical symptoms.

Acute Leukemia

Acute leukemia is further of two types, depending upon the type of malignant cell present: acute lymphoblastic leukemia (ALL) and acute myeloblastic leukemia (AML). In ALL, chromosomal translocation or abnormal chromosome numbers can lead to mutations in precursor lymphoid cells leading to lymphoblasts. Common mutations include t(12;21) and t(9;22). In AML, chromosomal translocations, rearrangements, and gain or loss of chromosomes can lead to mutations and abnormal production of myeloblasts. One important translocation is t(15;17), which leads to the fusion of retinoic acid receptor alpha (RARA) and a promyelocytic leukemia transcription factor (PML). This leads to the development of acute promyelocytic leukemia, which can present with hallmarks of disseminated intravascular coagulation and need emergent treatment with retinoic acid.

Chronic Leukemia

Like acute leukemia, even chronic leukemia is of two types: chronic lymphoblastic leukemia and chronic myeloblastic leukemia. The most common cause of chronic leukemia are the chromosomal abnormalities in hematopoietic stem cells that are precursors to leucocytes. Examples of such abnormalities are deletions, translocations, or extra-chromosomes. In CML, mutations mostly affect granulocytes (most commonly the t(9;22) translocation), and in CLL, they mostly affect lymphocytes (especially B lymphocytes). Unlike acute leukemia, in chronic leukemia, cells are partially mature. These partially mature cells do not function effectively and divide too quickly. They accumulate in the peripheral blood and lymphoid organs, which can lead to anemia and thrombocytopenia, and leukopenia.

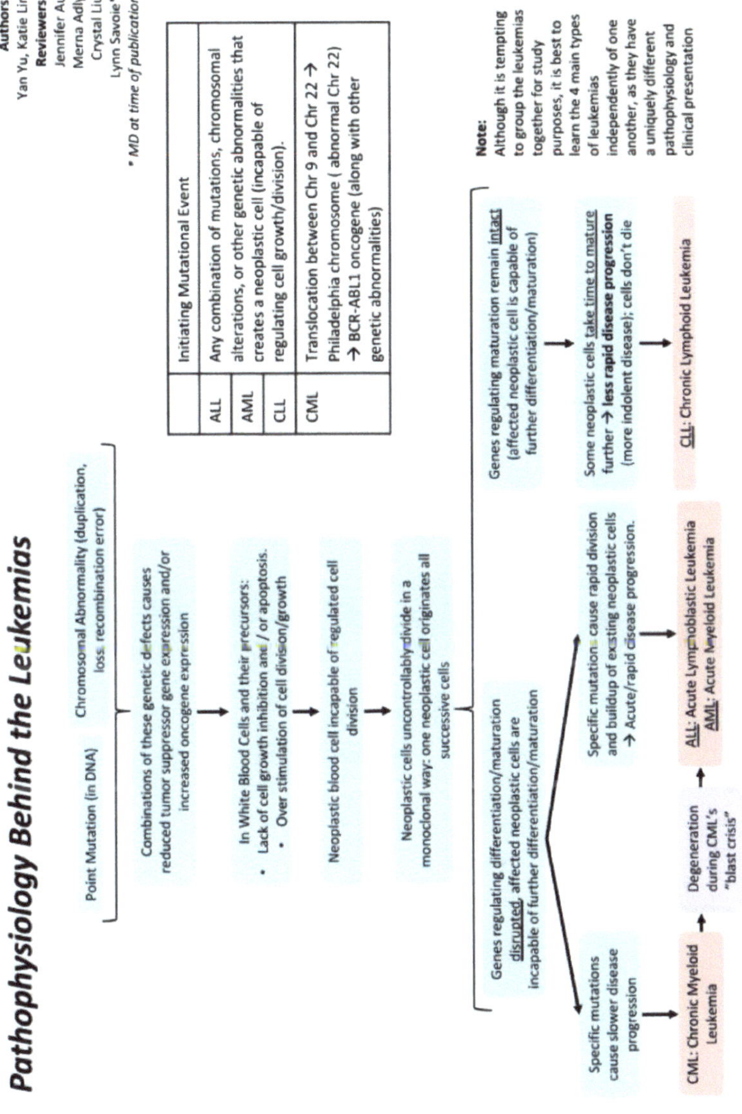

- **CLASSIFICATION**

A. Based on the clinical course of the disease and the type of cell line that is involved, leukemias are classified as:-

1. Acute Leukemia
   a. Acute Lymphoblastic leukemia (ALL)
   a. Acute Myeloblastic leukemia (AML)
2. Chronic Leukemia
   a. Chronic Lymphocytic leukemia (CLL)
   b. Chronic Myelocytic leukemia (CML)

B. FAB CLASSIFICATION OF ACUTE MYELOID LEUKEMIA

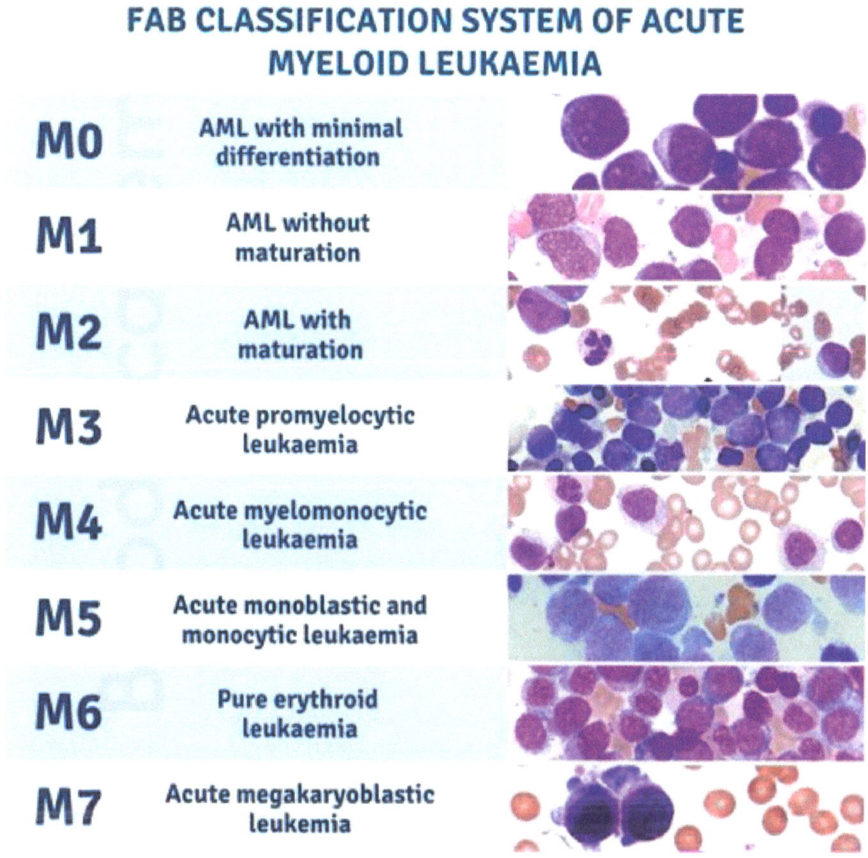

FAB CLASSIFICATION SYSTEM OF ACUTE MYELOID LEUKAEMIA

M0	AML with minimal differentiation
M1	AML without maturation
M2	AML with maturation
M3	Acute promyelocytic leukaemia
M4	Acute myelomonocytic leukaemia
M5	Acute monoblastic and monocytic leukaemia
M6	Pure erythroid leukaemia
M7	Acute megakaryoblastic leukemia

C. **WHO classification of myeloid neoplasms and acute leukemia**

a. Myeloproliferative neoplasms (MPN)

1. Chronic myeloid leukemia (CML), BCR-ABL
2. Chronic neutrophilic leukemia (CNL)
3. Polycythemia vera (PV)
4. Primary myelofibrosis (PMF) PMF, prefibrotic/early stage

PMF, overt fibrotic stage

5. Essential thrombocythemia (ET)
6. Chronic eosinophilic leukemia, not otherwise specified (NOS)
7. MPN, unclassifiable
8. Mastocytosis

b. Myeloid/lymphoid neoplasms with eosinophilia and rearrangement of PDGFRA, PDGFRB, or FGFR1, or with PCM1-JAK2

1. Myeloid/lymphoid neoplasms with PDGFRA rearrangement
2. Myeloid/lymphoid neoplasms with PDGFRB rearrangement
3. Myeloid/lymphoid neoplasms with FGFR1 rearrangement

Provisional entity: Myeloid/lymphoid neoplasms with PCM1-JAK2

c. Myelodysplastic/myeloproliferative neoplasms (MDS/MPN)

1. Chronic myelomonocytic leukemia (CMML)
2. Atypical chronic myeloid leukemia (aCML), BCR-ABL
3. Juvenile myelomonocytic leukemia (JMML)
4. MDS/MPN with ring sideroblasts and thrombocytosis (MDS/MPN-RS-T)
5. MDS/MPN, unclassifiable

d. Myelodysplastic syndromes (MDS)

1. MDS with single lineage dysplasia

2. MDS with ring sideroblasts (MDS-RS) MDS-RS and single lineage dysplasia

MDS-RS and multilineage dysplasia

3. MDS with multilineage dysplasia

4. MDS with excess blasts

5. MDS with isolated del(5q)

6. MDS, unclassifiable

Provisional entity: Refractory cytopenia of childhood

7. Myeloid neoplasms with germ line predisposition

e. Acute myeloid leukemia (AML) and related neoplasms

1. AML with recurrent genetic abnormalities

- AML with t(8;21)(q22;q22.1);RUNX1-RUNX1T1
- AML with inv(16)(p13.1q22) or t(16;16)(p13.1;q22);CBFB-MYH11
- APL with PML-RARA
- AML with t(9;11)(p21.3;q23.3);MLLT3-KMT2A
- AML with t(6;9)(p23;q34.1);DEK-NUP214
- AML with inv(3)(q21.3q26.2) or t(3;3)(q21.3;q26.2); GATA2, MECOM
- AML (megakaryoblastic) with t(1;22)(p13.3;q13.3);RBM15-MKL1
- *Provisional entity: AML with BCR-ABL1*
- AML with mutated NPM1

- AML with biallelic mutations of CEBPA
- *Provisional entity: AML with mutated RUNX1*

2. AML with myelodysplasia-related changes

3. Therapy-related myeloid neoplasms

4. AML, NOS

    - AML with minimal differentiation
    - AML without maturation
    - AML with maturation
    - Acute myelomonocytic leukemia
    - Acute monoblastic/monocytic leukemia
    - Pure erythroid leukemia
    - Acute megakaryoblastic leukemia
    - Acute basophilic leukemia
    - Acute panmyelosis with myelofibrosis

5. Myeloid sarcoma

6. Myeloid proliferations related to Down syndrome

    - Transient abnormal myelopoiesis (TAM)
    - Myeloid leukemia associated with Down syndrome

f. Blastic plasmacytoid dendritic cell neoplasm

g. Acute leukemias of ambiguous lineage

    1. Acute undifferentiated leukemia

    2. Mixed phenotype acute leukemia (MPAL) with t(9;22)(q34.1;q11.2); BCR- ABL1

    3. MPAL with t(v;11q23.3); KMT2A rearranged

    4. MPAL, B/myeloid, NOS

    5. MPAL, T/myeloid, NOS

h. B-lymphoblastic leukemia/lymphoma

    1. B-lymphoblastic leukemia/lymphoma, NOS

2. B-lymphoblastic leukemia/lymphoma with recurrent genetic abnormalities

3. B-lymphoblastic leukemia/lymphoma with t(9;22)(q34.1;q11.2);BCR- ABL1

4. B-lymphoblastic leukemia/lymphoma with t(v;11q23.3);KMT2A rearranged

5. B-lymphoblastic leukemia/lymphoma with t(12;21)(p13.2;q22.1); ETV6- RUNX1

6. B-lymphoblastic leukemia/lymphoma with hyperdiploidy

7. B-lymphoblastic leukemia/lymphoma with hypodiploidy

8. B-lymphoblastic leukemia/lymphoma with t(5;14)(q31.1;q32.3) IL3-IGH

9. B-lymphoblastic leukemia/lymphoma with t(1;19)(q23;p13.3);TCF3-PBX1

- *Provisional entity: B-lymphoblastic leukemia/lymphoma, BCR-ABL1–like*
- *Provisional entity: B-lymphoblastic leukemia/lymphoma with iAMP21*

i. T-lymphoblastic leukemia/lymphoma

- *Provisional entity: Early T-cell precursor lymphoblastic leukemia*
- *Provisionalentity: Natural killer (NK) cell lymphoblastic leukemia/ lymphoma*[78]

ORAL MANIFESTATIONS OF LEUKEMIA

Oral manifestation	Management
Gingival enlargement	Meticulous oral hygiene by use of soft bristle tooth brush
	Topical antiseptics (chlorhexidine 0.12% mouth rinse twice a day)
Oral ulcerations	Topical steroid (fluocinonide 0.05% gel) four times a day
	Antibiotic therapy is occasionally administered to prevent bacterial infection
	Biopsy if necessary
Noma and noma-like lesions	Antibiotic therapy
	Topical antiseptics (0.12% chlorhexidine mouth rinse twice a day)
	Oral hygiene
Myeloid sarcoma	Biopsy
	Antineoplastic therapy
Gingival bleeding	Meticulous oral hygiene by use of soft bristle tooth brush
	Antifibrinolytic mouth rinse
Oral, dental and periodontal infections	Infection foci removal (e.g. periodontal treatment, dental extractions)
	Topical antiseptics (chlorhexidine 0.12% mouth rinse twice a day)
	Antibiotics, antivirals and antifungals are administered to prevent and/or treat respectively bacterial, virus and fungal infections
	Granulocyte colony-stimulating factor is administered as an adjuvant
Trismus	Physiatrics

ACUTE MYELOID LEUKEMIA

General Manifestations of AML

1. Complications of pancytopenia (anemia, neutropenia, and thrombocytopenia), including
2. Weakness, and easy fatigue,
3. Infections of variable severity, and/ or
4. Hemorrhagic findings such as gingival bleeding, ecchymoses, epistaxis or menorrhagia.[79]

Oral manifestations

1. Mucosal pallor related to anemia.

2. Spontaneous bleeding and petechial hemorrhages of gingivae, palate, tongue or lips arising from thrombocytopenia.

3. Gingival hyperplasia caused by leukemic infiltration.

4. Oral ulcerations are frequent and may follow either neutropenia or direct infiltration by leukemic cells.

5. Patients may exhibit recurrent viral, bacterial, and fungal infections (like herpes and candidiasis) as a consequence of immunosuppression.[80]
6. Atypical features such as chin numbness, tooth pain and mobility, cracked lips and hemorrhagic bullae on the anterior dorsum of the tongue, buccal and labial mucosa.[79]
7. Rare oral manifestation associated with AML is the noma-like lesion.[81]

The most prevalent oral signs and symptoms are:

- Gingival bleeding,

- Oral ulceration (fig no. 2 a and b)

- Gingival hyperplasia. (fig no. 2 c and d)

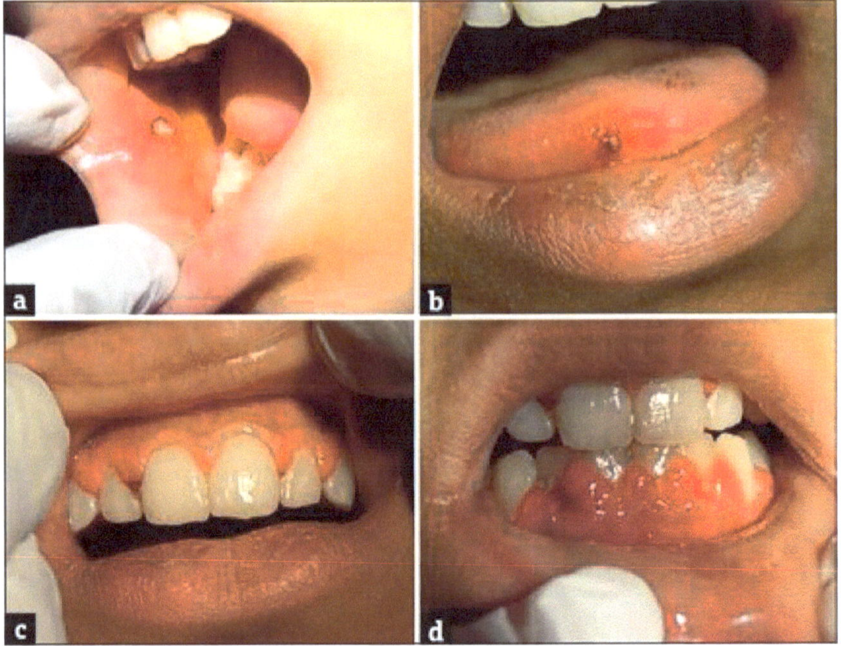

Fig. No. .2

CHRONIC MYELOID LEUKEMIA

Oral Manifestations of CML

1. Bleeding gums
2. Gingival enlargements and
3. Mucosal tissue enlargement from direct leukemic cell infiltration.
4. Granulocytic sarcoma of the jaws.[82]

ACUTE LYMPHOBLASTIC LEUKEMIA General manifestations of ALL

1. Pancytopenia (anemia, neutropenia or thrombocytopenia)

2. Fatigue
3. Dyspnea
4. Fever
5. Pallor
6. Weight loss
7. Bleeding.
8. Hepatosplenomegaly
9. Lymphadenopathy
10. Bone pain.

Oral manifestations of ALL

1. Mucosal pallor
2. Gingival bleeding
3. Echymoses
4. lymphadenopathy of the head and neck region[83]
5. Pericoronitis[84]
6. Trismus[85]
7. Mucosal anomalies
    - extensive ulcers

- coated tongue
- fetor oris
- shallow papillae
- tender oral mucosa and
- oral mucosal infections (mucositis, candidiasis, herpes simplex, varicella/zoster and cytomegalovirus)[86]

CHRONIC LYMPHOBLASTIC LEUKEMIA

Oral manifestations of CLL

1. Local swelling, with or without ulceration and pain.
2. Recurrent oral bleeding.
3. Purpura and gingival bleeding
4. Recurrent epistaxis and asymptomatic intraoral swelling
5. Isolated, intermittent, and severe nosebleeds
6. Palatal enlargement
7. Gingival leukemic infiltration.[83]

- <u>DENTAL MANAGEMENT</u>

GENERAL CONSIDERATIONS REGARDING DENTAL TREATMENT

1. Multidisciplinary approach involving oncologists, nurses, dentists (general and stomatological practitioners), social workers, nutritionists, and other health professionals.

2. The classification of patients into categories of high, moderate, and low risk for dental treatment, based on the type of leukemia (acute or chronic) and chemotherapy.

    - **High risk group:** those with active leukemia, high number of neoplastic cells in the bone marrow and peripheral blood; they are thrombocytopenic and neutropenic. antileukemic patients under treatment, present bone marrow suppression.

    - **Moderate risk group**: successfully completed the first phase of treatment (induction) and are undergoing the maintenance phase, no sign of malignancy in the bone marrow or peripheral blood; present myelosuppression due to chemotherapy.

    - **Low-risk group**: successfully completed treatment and present no evidence of malignancy or myelosuppression.

3. Basic health care should be part of the patient's routine.

    Objectives of care include

    - prevention of infection, pain control, maintenance of oral functions, and management of complications of antineoplastic therapy, aimed at improving the quality of life of patients.[87]

Little et al.[88] reinforce that the role of the dentist should occur at three different moments:

1. Pre-antineoplastic treatment evaluation and preparation of patients for this

2. Guidelines and oral health care during treatment

3. Post-treatment care

PRE-ANTINEOPLASTIC TREATMENT EVALUATION AND PATIENT PREPARATION

The objectives of the pre-antineoplastic treatment dental evaluation are as follows:[89]

1. Identify and eliminate sources of existing or potential infection, without, however, promoting complications or delaying cancer therapy.

2. Educate the patient (or their relatives) about the importance of maintaining oral health in reducing problems and oral discomfort before, during, and after cancer treatment.

3. Warn about the possible effects of antineoplastic therapy in the oral cavity, such as mucositis.

4. Identify specific issues of the diagnosis of leukemia, such as leukemic infiltrates in oral tissues.

ORAL HEALTH CARE DURING ANTINEOPLASTIC TREATMENT

The objectives of dental care during chemotherapy are as follows:

1. Maintain optimal oral health

2. Treat side effects of antineoplastic therapy

3. Reinforce to the patient the importance of oral health in reducing problems/discomforts arising from chemotherapy.

POST-ANTINEOPLASTIC TREATMENT ORAL HEALTH

In the post-antineoplastic treatment phase, patients are considered cured of leukemia and not having oral manifestations due to illness or chemotherapy, except for those with sequelae of radiotherapy or children who received chemotherapy in the stage of tooth formation, which may present hypoplastic areas on tooth enamel (mineralization disorder) and changes in the development of dental roots (which are presented short and V-shaped).[89]

DENTAL PROCEDURES IN DIFFERENT STAGES OF THE DISEASE AND TREATMENT

Dental treatment should be planned according to the anti-neoplastic therapy and Hematopoetic Stem-Cell Transplantation (HSCT). The execution of some dental procedures especially those of invasive character depends on the overall health status of the patient and stage of antineoplastic treatment in which it lies.

a. Dental Treatment in the Prechemotherapy Phase

Procedure	Considerations and restrictions	Time before the start of CT
Type I		
Exam Clinical Radiographic Hygiene instructions	No restrictions.	–
Molding	Elective procedure, postpone	–
Type II		
Simple restorations (ART) Prophylaxis and supragingival scaling	No restrictions.	–
Orthodontics	Elective treatment, postpone. Consider removing orthodontic appliances.	–
Type III		
More complex restorations	Solely for adequacy of the oral environment. Consider use of provisional restorative materials (e.g., glass ionomer).	–
Scaling and root planning (subgingival)	Invasive procedure of high-risk carried out carefully. To evaluate hematological indices of platelets and neutrophils. Need for antibiotic prophylaxis.	–
Endodontics		
Symptomatic tooth	Evaluate hematological indices of platelets and neutrophils. Need for antibiotic prophylaxis. Consider extraction if endodontics fail.	At least 1 week [1]
Asymptomatic tooth	Postpone (tricresol formalin) OR Evaluate hematological indices of platelets and neutrophils. Need for antibiotic prophylaxis.	At least 1 week [1]
Type IV		
Simple extractions	Invasive procedure of high-risk. Evaluate hematological indices of platelets and neutrophils. Need for antibiotic prophylaxis.	3 weeks; minimum 10–14 days [5] 2 weeks; minimum 7–10 days [1]
Curettage (gingivoplasty)	Elective procedure, invasive and high-risk. Postpone.	–
Type V		
Multiple extractions	If for adequacy of the oral environment, evaluate hematological indices of platelets and neutrophils. Need for antibiotic prophylaxis. If elective, postpone.	3 weeks; minimum 10–14 days [5] 2 weeks; minimum 7–10 days [1]
Flap surgery/gingivectomy Extraction of impacted tooth Apicoectomy Single implant placement	Elective procedure, invasive and high-risk. Postpone.	–
Type VI		
Extraction of an entire arch or both	If adequacy of the oral environment, evaluate hematological indices of platelets and neutrophils. Need for antibiotic prophylaxis. If elective, postpone.	3 weeks; minimum 10–14 days [5] 2 weeks; minimum 7–10 days [1]
Extraction of multiple impacted teeth Flap surgery Orthognathic surgery Placement of multiple implants	Elective procedure, invasive and high-risk. Postpone.	–

b. Dental Treatment in the Transchemotherapy Phase.

Procedure	Considerations or restrictions	Time between cycles
Type I		
Exam		
Clinical Radiographic Hygiene instructions	No restrictions.	—
Molding	Elective procedure. Postpone.	—
Type II		
Simple restorations (ART) Prophylaxis and supragingival scaling	No restrictions.	—
Orthodontics	Elective treatment. Consider removing orthodontic appliances.	—
Type III		
More complex restorations	Solely for adequacy of the oral environment. Consider use of provisional restorative materials (eg., Glass ionomer).	—
Scaling and root planning (subgingival)	Invasive treatment, of high-risk, perform carefully. Evaluate hematological indices of platelets and neutrophils. Need for antibiotic prophylaxis.	—
Endodontics		
Symptomatic tooth	Evaluate hematological indices of platelets and neutrophils. Need for antibiotic prophylaxis. Consider extraction if endodontics fails.	At least 1 week [1]
Asymptomatic tooth	Postpone (tricresol formalin). OR Evaluate hematological indices of platelets and neutrophils. Need for antibiotic prophylaxis.	At least 1 week [1]
Type IV		
Simple extractions	Invasive treatment of high-risk. Evaluate hematological indices of platelets and neutrophils. Need for antibiotic prophylaxis.	3 weeks; minimum 10–14 days [5] 2 weeks; minimum 7–10 days [1]
Curettage (gingivoplasty)	Elective treatment, invasive and high-risk. Postpone.	—
Type V		
Multiple extractions	If adequacy of the oral environment, evaluate hematological indices of platelets and neutrophils. Need for antibiotic prophylaxis. If elective, postpone.	3 weeks; minimum 10–14 days [5] 2 weeks; minimum 7–10 days [1]
Flap surgery/gingivectomy Extraction of impacted tooth Apicoectomy Single implant placement	Elective procedure, invasive and high-risk. Postpone.	—
Type VI		
Extraction of an entire arch or both	If adequacy of the oral environment, evaluate hematological indices of platelets and neutrophils. Need for antibiotic prophylaxis. If elective, postpone.	3 weeks; minimum 10–14 days [5] 2 weeks; minimum 7–10 days [1]
Extraction of multiple impacted teeth Flap surgery Orthognathic surgery Placement of multiple implants	Elective procedure, invasive and high-risk. Postpone.	—

c. Dental Treatment after Chemotherapy

Intervention in postchemotherapy	Considerations and restrictions
Type I	
Exam	
Clinic	
Radiographic	No restrictions.
Hygiene instructions	
Molding	
Type II	
Simple restorations (ART)	No restrictions.
Prophylaxis and supragingival cell scaling	
Orthodontics	Completed chemotherapy and after two years free of disease, one can restart the orthodontic treatment
Type III	
More complex restorations	
Scaling and root planning cell (subgingival)	
Endodontics	No restrictions.
Symptomatic tooth	
Asymptomatic tooth	
Type IV	
Simple extractions	Need for antibiotic prophylaxis until six months after completion of chemotherapy.
Curettage (gingivoplasty)	
Type V	
Multiple extractions	
Flap surgery/gingivectomy	
Extraction of impacted tooth	Need for antibiotic prophylaxis until six months after completion of chemotherapy.
Apicoectomy	
Single implant placement	
Type VI	
Extraction of an entire arch or both	
Extraction of multiple impacted cell teeth	
Flap surgery	Need for antibiotic prophylaxis until six months after completion of chemotherapy.
Orthognathic surgery	
Placement of multiple implants	

- **DENTAL COMPLICATIONS**

Multi agent chemotherapy and radiation therapy have greatly increased the chances of survival and are widely accepted. However, these treatment modalities lead to oral complications and have an impact on the developing dentition and on orofacial growth.[91]

1. Oral mucositis (OM) is the most common oral complications that follow chemotherapy and radiotherapy.
2. Change in quality and quantity of saliva due to anticancer treatment.[92]

3. Increase in the number of dental anomalies such as agenesis, microdontia, tapering roots and short roots, affect the dental age maturity.

4. For pediatric patients who are undergoing bone marrow transplant and radiotherapy, they may develop graft-versus-host disease (GVHD) after the transplantation approximately by 2-3 weeks, and it is induced by the cytotoxic effect of the donor T lymphocytes in the receiver tissues. Those patients may manifest oral signs such as: erythema, erosion, ulceration of the mucosa, lichenoid changes, and xerostomia.[93]
5. Oral complications of treatment of leukemia in children such as leukemic infiltration in the mandible, trismus, mucormycosis and oral aspergillosis.[94]

(B.) LYMPHOMAS & RETICULOENDOTHELIAL NEOPLASMS

- INTRODUCTION
- ETIOLOGY
- PATHOPHYSIOLOGY
- CLASSIFICATION
- ORAL MANIFESTATIONS
- DENTAL MANAGEMENT
- DENTAL COMPLICATIONS

• INTRODUCTION

Cancers that develop in the lymph system are called the Lymphomas. A watery like fluid called the lymph is carried in this system. It contains white blood cells, or lymphocytes. This network is a key part of the body's immune system. The lymphatic system helps filter out dead cells and other debris from the bloodstream. It also helps protect the body against germs, including bacteria and viruses. There are many parts of lymphatic system. These include the spleen, tonsils and adenoids, thymus and lymph nodes ("glands") in the neck, underarms, stomach and groin. Lymph vessels connect these organs and nodes together. Once a malignancy begins in one part of the lymph system, it often spreads throughout the rest of the system before it is detected.

Lymphomas (Hodgkin and non-Hodgkin lymphoma) are the third most common cancer in children, but it is still rare. They present with symptoms such as painless swelling of the lymph nodes, fever and fatigue. According to the cell types that make up the cancer, lymphomas are divided into sub-groups. They are classified as either non-Hodgkin's and Hodgkin's. Of these two types, non-Hodgkin's (NHL) is the more common lymphoma in children, and it occurs more frequently between the ages of 10 and 20 than under ten. Approximately 6-7% of cancers in children are NHL type. Whereas the Hodgkin's is rare in children under five years of age. In children under age 10, it is more common in boys than in girls.

There are many types of lymphoma but only four common subtypes of lymphoma are encountered in children:

- Burkitt and Burkitt-like lymphoma
- Diffuse large B-cell lymphoma
- Anaplastic large cell lymphoma
- Lymphoblastic lymphoma (of B- or T-cell origin)[95]

- **ETIOLOGY**

Researchers have found some factors that can increase a child's risk of NHL. But most children with NHL do not have any known risk factors that can be changed.

1. Age, gender, and race

Non-Hodgkin lymphoma is rare in children in general, but it is more common in older children than in younger ones. It is also more common in boys than in girls and in White children than in Black children. The reasons for these gender and racial differences are not clear.

2. Having a weakened immune system

Some types of immune system problems have been linked with a higher risk of NHL in children and teens.

3. Congenital (present at birth) immune deficiency syndromes

Some children are born with an abnormal immune system because of a genetic (inherited) syndrome. Along with an increased risk of serious infections, these children also have a higher risk of developing NHL (and sometimes other cancers as well). These syndromes include:

- Wiskott-Aldrich syndrome
- Nijmegen syndrome
- Ataxia-telangiectasia
- Common variable immunodeficiency
- X-linked lymphoproliferative syndrome

4. Organ transplant

Children who have had organ transplants are treated with drugs that weaken their immune system to prevent it from attacking the new organ. These children have an increased risk of developing NHL that is almost always caused by Epstein-Barr virus infection (see below). The risk depends on which drugs and what doses are used.

5. Human immunodeficiency virus (HIV) infection and AIDS

Infection with HIV, the virus that causes AIDS, can weaken the immune system. Children with HIV generally get the infection from contact with their mother's blood, usually before or during birth. Because HIV infection is a risk factor for developing NHL, doctors may recommend that children with NHL be tested for HIV infection.

6. Epstein-Barr virus infection

In areas of Africa where Burkitt lymphoma is common, chronic infection with both malaria and the Epstein-Barr virus (EBV) is an important risk factor. EBV has been linked with almost all Burkitt lymphomas in Africa.

EBV infection is life-long, although it doesn't cause serious problems in most people. In Americans who are first infected with EBV as teens or young adults, it can cause infectious mononucleosis, sometimes known simply as mono. Most Americans have been infected with EBV by the time they are adults, but the infection seems to occur later in life in the United States than in Africa, which may help explain why it is less likely to cause childhood lymphoma here. Exactly how EBV is linked to NHL is not completely understood, but it seems to have to do with the ability of the virus to infect and alter B lymphocytes.

7. Radiation exposure

Radiation exposure may be a minor risk factor in childhood NHL. Survivors of atomic bomb exposures and nuclear reactor accidents have an increased risk of developing some types of cancer. Leukemia and thyroid cancers are the most common, but there is a slightly increased risk of NHL as well.

Patients treated with radiation therapy for other cancers have a slightly increased risk of NHL later in life. But it usually takes many years for this to develop, so these secondary cases of NHL are more common in adults than in children.

The possible risks from fetal or childhood exposure to lower levels of radiation, such as from x-ray tests or CT scans, are not known for sure. If there is an increase in risk for NHL or other cancers it is likely to be small, but to be safe, most doctors recommend that pregnant women and children not get these tests unless they are absolutely needed.

8. Other possible risk factors

Some research has suggested that a family history of NHL (in a brother, sister, or parent) might raise the risk of lymphoma. Lymphoma risk may also be higher in children of older mothers. More research is needed to confirm these findings, but if there is an increased risk tied to these factors, it is likely to be small.[96]

PATHOPHYSIOLOGY (fig. no. 3)

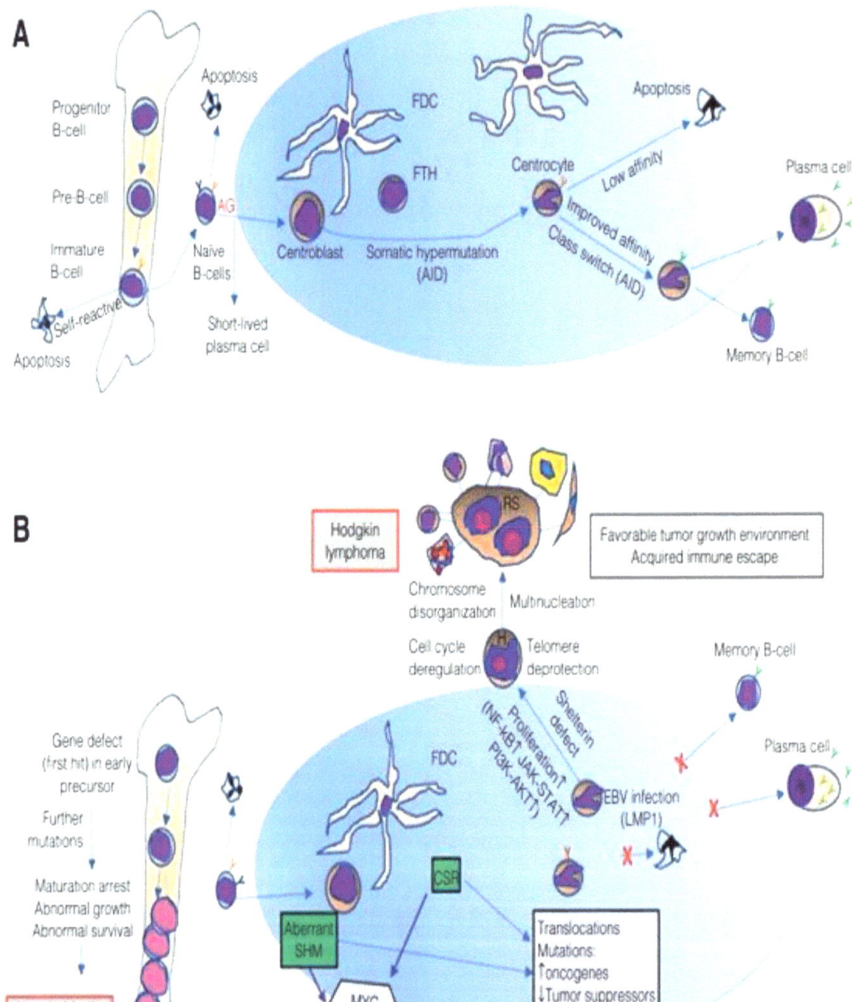

FIGURE 3: Normal B-cell development and simplified pathogenesis of B-cell lymphomas.

A. B-cells develop and mature in the bone marrow where B-cell receptor (BCR) gene is rearranged and BCR is counter-selected for autoreactivity (eliminated by apoptosis if self-reactive). The positively selected B cells become mature naive B cells that leave the bone marrow. Upon encountering cognate antigen, some activated B cells differentiate into short-lived plasma cells secreting low- affinity antibodies and providing a rapid initial response to the antigen. Some activated B cells migrate into lymphoid follicles and initiate a germinal center (GC), where GC-B cells go through somatic hypermutation (SHM) and class switch recombination (CSR), both of which are dependent on the activity of activation-induced cytidine deaminase (AID). After several cycles of proliferation, mutation, and positive selection, GC-B cells differentiate into either high-affinity antibody-secreting plasma cells or memory B cells and leave the GC.

B. With further mutations, the B-cell precursors with gene defect gain dysregulated signals of growth, survival and differentiation, and eventually develop into B- lymphoblastic lymphoma. The DNA modification processes of GC-B cells make them prone to chromosome translocations and mutations. The GC-B cells with translocation involving *MYC* gene and deregulated signal pathways of growth and survival eventually develop into Burkitt lymphoma. With additional genetic lesions, GC-B cells with translocations and/or mutations involving other oncogenes and/or tumor suppressor genes develop into diffuse large B-cell lymphoma of GC-B type. GC-B cells with deregulated NF-κB pathway driven by EBV proto-oncogene LMP1 in EBV+ cases or certain mutations in EBV- cases develop into Hodgkin (H) cells. Chromosome disorganization and multinucleation due to cell cycle deregulation and telomere deprotection lead H cells to develop into Reed-Steinberg (RS) cells. The H and RS cells further their survival by attracting a supportive microenvironment through releasing cytokines and growth factors and suppressing local immune response. Eventually Hodgkin lymphoma is developed. ↑- increased signaling or activity; x-inhibited process.

Hodgkin lymphoma results from the clonal transformation of cells of B-cell origin, giving rise to pathognomic binucleated Reed-Sternberg cells.

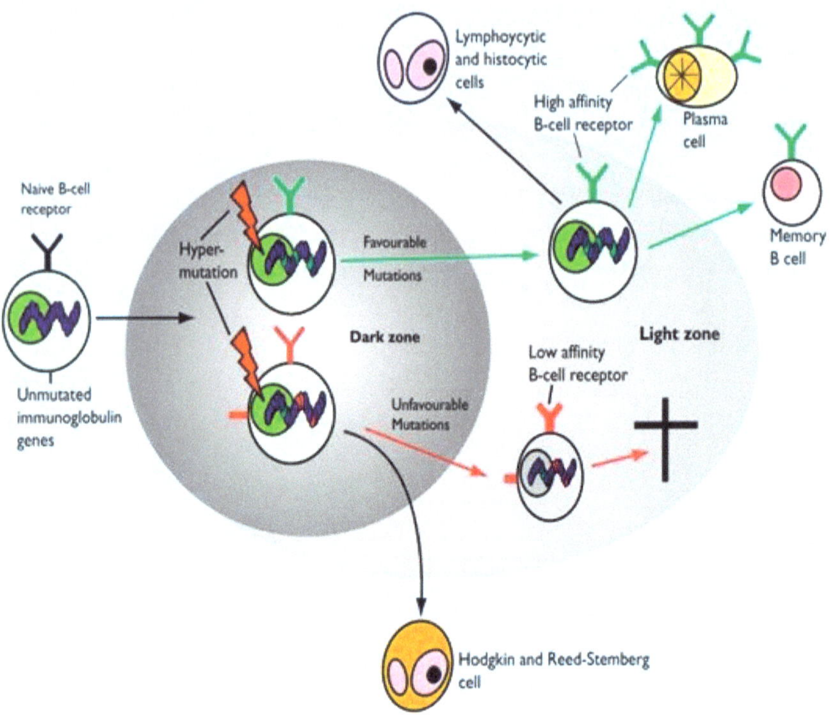

FIGURE 4 : Pathogenesis of Hodgkin lymphoma.

The germinal-center derivation of Hodgkin and Reed-Stemberg cells in classic Hodgkin lymphoma and lymphomatic and histiocytic cells in noduler lymphocyte-predominant Hodgkin lymphoma.

Hodgkin-Reed-Sternberg (H-RS) cells are the diagnostic tumor cell in classic HL. It is believed that the H-RS cells are derived in the germinal center and that they have clonally rearranged but crippled immunoglobulin genes (unfavorable mutations), which lead them to inhibition of apoptosis (programmed cell death) and lead to systemic lymphoma disease. 23,27 The cells have lost their capacity to express a high-affinity B-cell receptor (Figure 4) and escape negative selection. Several aberrantly activated signaling pathways and transcription factors have been identified that contribute to the rescue of HR-S cells from apoptosis.23,24,27 Recent studies show that B cells enter the germinal center with an activated FAS-mediated apoptosis. It is believed that execution of apoptosis is prevented in germinal center B cells by up-regulation of an inhibitor called c-FLIP (an inhibitor of FAS-mediated apoptosis).27,28 Also high levels of the nuclear transcription factor-– (NF-) have been found in H-RS cells; these high NF- levels may play a role in pathogenesis by interfering with apoptosis.24,28EBV is linked to the development of HL because it is believed that EBV possesses a transforming ability that leads to NF- activation in antigen-activated B cells.29

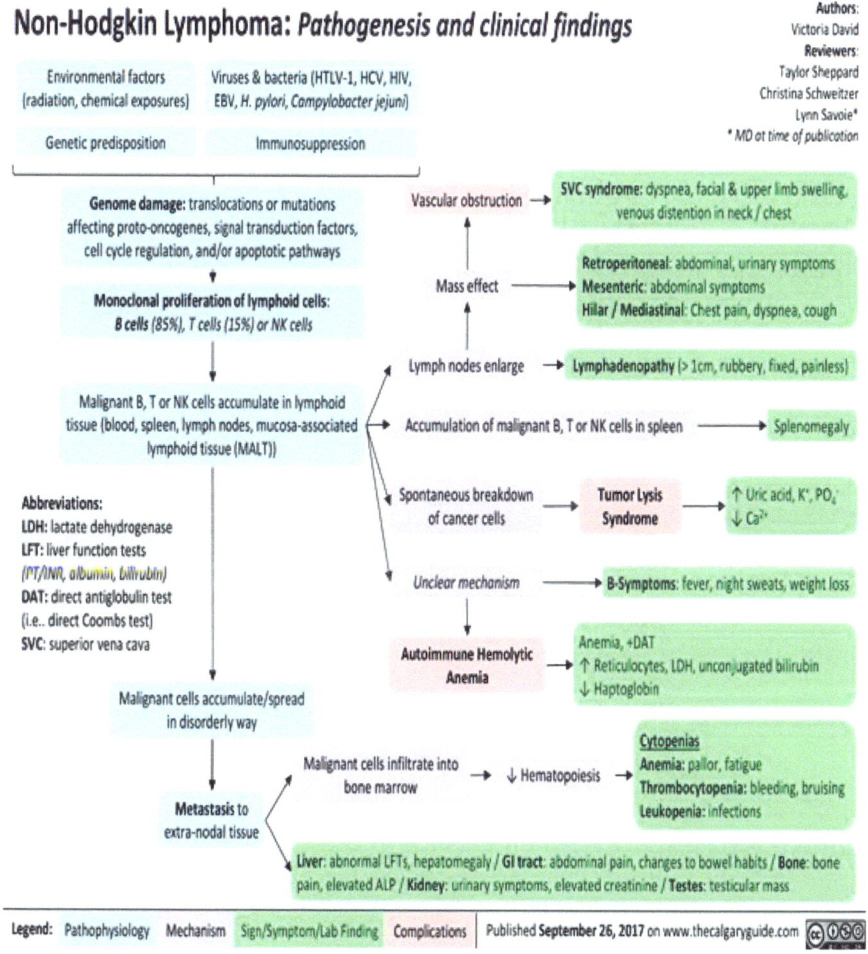

Figure 5: Etiopathogenesis and clinical features of non Hodgkin lymphoma.

- **CLASSIFICATION**

Twenty-five years after the Revised European American Classification of Lymphoid Neoplasms classification was published, its principle of an integrative approach to disease definition based on several parameters still prevails and has been adopted and expanded in the following World Health Organization classifications of tumors of the hematopoietic organs. The latest World Health Organization classification revised in 2017 comprises more than 80 entities of mature lymphoid neoplasms (B-cell, T-cell, and Hodgkin lymphomas), which are defined according to their morphology, immunophenotype, genetic lesions and molecular profiles, clinical features, and cellular derivation. The classification also recognizes both incipient and indolent lymphoid neoplasms with a low potential of progression.[97]

2017 WHO Classification of Mature Lymphomas B-Cell Neoplasms

Predominantly disseminated

- Chronic lymphocytic leukemia/B-cell small lymphocytic lymphoma
- Monoclonal B-cell lymphocytosis,
- B-cell prolymphocytic leukemia
- Splenic marginal zone B-cell lymphoma
- Hairy cell leukemia
- Splenic B-cell lymphoma/leukemia, unclassifiable*

- Splenic diffuse red pulp small B-cell lymphoma*
- Hairy cell leukemia—variant*
- Lymphoplasmacytic lymphoma
- Waldenström macroglobulinemia
- Monoclonal gammopathy of unknown significance (MGUS) immunoglobulin
- Mu heavy-chain disease
- Gamma heavy-chain disease
- Alpha heavy-chain disease
- MGUS immunoglobulin G/A+
- Plasma cell myeloma
- Solitary plasmacytoma of bone
- Extraosseous plasmacytoma
- Monoclonal immunoglobulin deposition disease

Primary extranodal or nodal

- Extranodal marginal zone B-cell lymphoma of mucosa-associated lymphoid tissue
- Nodal marginal zone B-cell lymphoma Pediatric nodal marginal zone lymphoma*

- Follicular lymphoma In situ follicular neoplasia Duodenal-type follicular lymphoma
- Pediatric-type follicular lymphoma
- Large B-cell lymphoma with IRF4 rearrangement*
- Primary cutaneous follicle center lymphoma
- Mantle cell lymphoma In situ mantle cell neoplasia
- DLBCL-NOS Germinal center B-cell type Activated B-cell type
- T-cell/histiocyte-rich large B-cell lymphoma
- Primary DLBCL of the central nervous system
- Primary cutaneous DLBCL, leg-type
- EBV+ DLBCL-NOS
- EBV+ mucocutaneous ulcer
- DLBCL associated with chronic inflammation
- Lymphomatoid granulomatosis
- Mediastinal (thymic) large B-cell lymphoma
- Intravascular large B-cell lymphoma
- ALK+ large B-cell lymphoma
- Plasmablastic lymphoma
- Primary effusion lymphoma
- HHV8+ DLBCL-NOS*

- Burkitt lymphoma
- Burkitt-like lymphoma with 11q aberration*
- Lymphomatoid granulomatosis
- High-grade B-cell lymphoma with MYC and BCL2 and/or BCL6 gene rearrangements*
- High-grade B-cell lymphoma NOS*
- B-cell lymphoma unclassifiable with features intermediate between DLBCL and cHL

T and NK-cell Neoplasms

Predominantly disseminated

- T-cell prolymphocytic leukemia
- T-cell large granular lymphocytic leukemia
- Aggressive NK-cell leukemia
- Chronic lymphoproliferative disorder of NK cells*
- Systemic EBV-positive T-cell lymphoma of childhood*
- Chronic active EBV infection of T- and NK-cell type, systemic form
- Adult T-cell lymphoma/leukemia (HTLV-1+)

Primary extranodal

- Extranodal NK/T-cell lymphoma, nasal type
- EATL
- Monomorphic epitheliotropic intestinal T-cell lymphoma
- Indolent T-cell lymphoproliferative disorder of the gastro-intestinal tract*
- Hepatosplenic T-cell lymphoma
- Subcutaneous panniculitis-like T-cell lymphoma
- Breast implant–associated ALCL*
- Subcutaneous panniculitis-like T-cell lymphoma

Primary cutaneous

- Mycosis fungoides
- Sézary syndrome
- Primary cutaneous CD30+ lymphoproliferative disorders

Lymphomatoid papulosis Primary cutaneous ALCL

- Primary cutaneous γδ T-cell lymphoma
- Provisional CD4+ or CD8+ entities*
- Hydroa vacciniforme–like lymphoproliferative disorder

- Severe mosquito bite allergy

Predominantly nodal

- PTCL-NOS
- Angioimmunoblastic T-cell lymphoma
- Follicular T-cell lymphoma
- Nodal PTCL with T follicular helper phenotype
- ALCL, ALK-positive
- ALCL, ALK-negative

Hodgkin lymphomas
Nodular lymphocyte predominance HL Classical HL

- Nodular sclerosis cHL
- Mixed cellularity cHL
- Lymphocyte-rich cHL
- Lymphocyte-depleted cHL

Immunodeficiency-associated lymphoproliferative disorders

- Post-transplantation lymphoproliferative disorders (PTLD)
- Nondestructive PTLD

- Plasmacytic hyperplasia
- Infectious mononucleosis PTLD
- Florid follicular hyperplasia PTLD
- Polymorphic PTLD
- Monomorphic PTLD
- cHL PTLD
- Other iatrogenic immunodeficiency-associated lymphoproliferative disorders

- <u>ORAL MANIFESTATIONS</u>

1. Hard tissue lesions:

Jaw bones: Appear as expansive lesions of jaws causing facial asymmetry. Bone changes in lymphoma may be because of the release of osteoclast-activating factors from the lymphoid cells. Endemic type (African) Burkitt's lymphoma involves the jaws in over 50% of cases.[98] (Fig no. 6)

Tooth and alveolar bone: When an osteolytic lesion of jaw involves the tooth they were reported to be mobile. Alveolar bone loss with oedema and pain may also occur which often mimics periodontal diseases. (Fig no. 7)

Temporo Mandibular Joint: There was only one case of jaw pain and trismus reported Alexiev et al.[99] In 2007 due to destruction of condyle by histiocytic sarcoma.

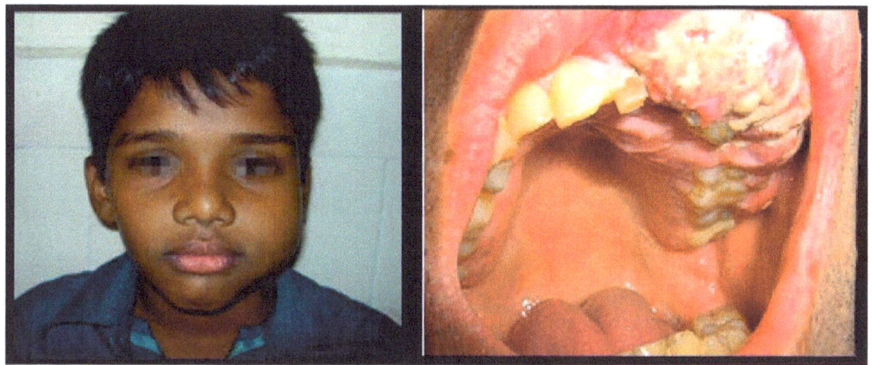

(Fig no. 6) (Fig no. 7)

2. Soft tissue lesions:

Soft tissue mass: Asymptomatic soft swelling with or without ulceration that primarily affect the tonsils, palate, buccal mucosa, gums, tongue, floor of the mouth, salivary glands, and retro molar region. Large B cell lymphoma cases have also been reported to present as Gingival and palatal mass. The palatal mass was also associated with ulcerated tissue with destruction of the bone and exposed dental roots, extending to the vestibular area of maxilla. (Fig no. 8)

Ulcers: Unlike myeloid malignancies lymphomas are not commonly presented as ulcers. If present they may be present as ulceration of surface of swellings. Mycosis fungoides can also appear as depressed ulcer.[100] (Fig no. 9)

Mucosal lesions: Mycosis fungiods is can appear as erythematous patches or plaques involving palate and tongue. Oral hairy leukoplakia an asymptomatic, corrugated white patch like lesion on the lateral borders of tongue was reported by Davis et al secondary to hairy cell leukoplakia. The lesion was reported to be due EBV infection and the location of the lesion was due to constant contact of resting tongue by EBV infected saliva.[101]

Lymph nodes: Non pain full enlargement of waldeyer's ring, tonsil and salivary gland lymph nodes has been reported. (Fig no. 10)

Salivary glands: Among tumors of the parotid lymphomas present 1% to 4% of cases. They are either extra nodal in origin or due to secondary replacement of parotid parenchyma by nodal lymphomas. Mantle cell lymphoma accounts for 3% of salivary gland tumours. Plasma cell myeloma of submandibular salivary gland was reported to be presented as non-tender upper neck swelling without any mass.

Neurologic manifestations: Numbness and paraesthesia has been reported in NHL, HL plasma cell myeloma and Histiocytic sarcoma.

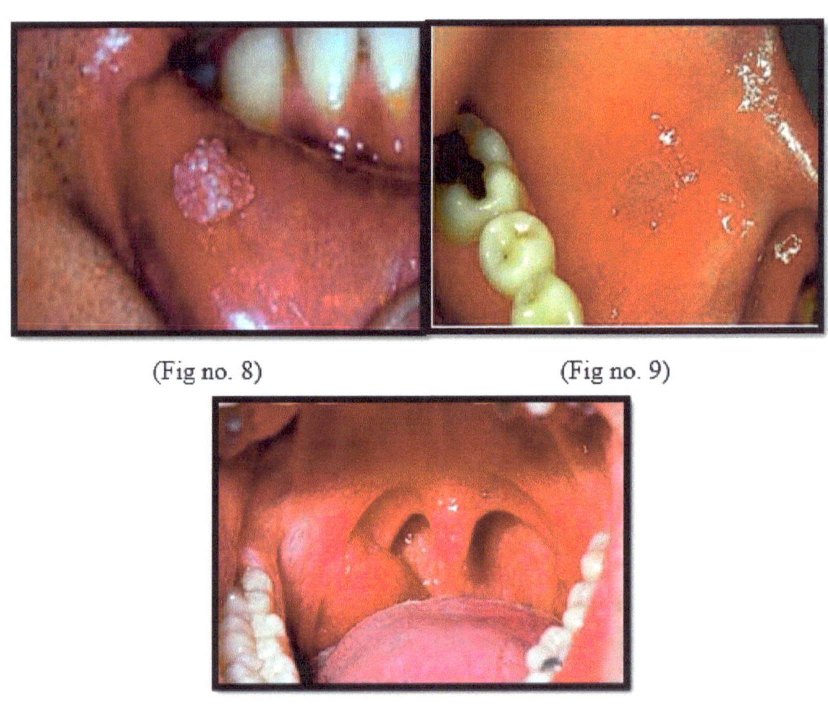

(Fig no. 8) (Fig no. 9)

(Fig no. 10)

- **DENTAL MANAGEMENT**

Treatment depends on the type and stage of lymphoma, signs and symptoms of the disease, availability of treatment, and the age and general health of the patient. The main aim of treatment is to achieve complete remission from the lymphoma. Different types of lymphoma respond differently, and therefore a variety of treatment options is necessary.

Hodgkin's lymphoma responds well to chemotherapeutic agents. On the other hand, low-grade non-Hodgkin's lymphoma is considered to be one of the most radiosensitive tumours, therefore it is usually treated with a low dose of radiotherapy (typically 36.6 Gray). Chemotherapy can also be added during the treatment of highgrade NHL. In both types of lymphoma, monoclonal antibodies may be added to chemotherapy cycles and can also be used for radioimmunotherapy. Other types of treatments might be considered, which will be detailed later in the paper.

Treatment types

The main treatment modalities for patients with lymphoma are:

1. Monoclonal antibodies (MABs);
2. Chemotherapy;
3. Radiotherapy;
4. Corticosteroid;
5. Haematopoietic stem cell transplant (HSCT).

DENTAL RECOMMENDATIONS FOR PATIENT UNDERGOIMG MONOCLONAL ANTIBODIES TREATMENT

- A dental assessment by the general dental practitioner (GDP) prior to starting a monoclonal antibody (generally rituximab) therapy is recommended to ensure that they are dentally fit prior to starting lymphoma treatment. This may involve extraction of infected or unrestorable teeth, or teeth with advanced periodontal disease. This should be carried out as soon as possible, and in liaison with a special care dentist or oral surgeon and the haemato-oncologist.
- It is rare for patients who are being treated with rituximab to develop medication-related osteonecrosis of the jaw (MRONJ), however it has been reported in literature.[102]

DENTAL RECOMMENDATIONS FOR PATIENT UNDERGOING CHEMOTHERAPY TREATMENT

- If pre-treatment extractions have not been possible, any necessary extractions should be planned in liaison with a patient's haemato-oncologist to determine the right time so as to reduce the risk of infection and aid haemostasis. It is important to ensure that there is sufficient time post-extraction (typically 10–14 days) to allow adequate healing prior to the next cycle of chemotherapy. Therefore, if the extraction is not urgent, it would be better to wait until after chemotherapy cycles are complete, and manage any dental infection through pulp extirpation and/or antibiotics.

- Dental extractions or regional block injection (ie inferior alveolar nerve block) should be avoided for patients with platelet counts below 50 x 109 /L and 30 x 109 /L, respectively.

- Ideally, dental treatment should be carried out within 24 hours from when the platelet transfusion has been given.

- A post-transfusion blood test is recommended to check that the platelets are at the required level as some patients do not increment as well as others.

- Local haemostatic measures are recommended, such as the use of haemostatic agents (Surgicel®) suturing the socket, as well as written and verbal post- operative instructions and the provision of an emergency contact.

- Scully et al recommend antibiotic prophylaxis for patients with neutrophil counts below 2 x 109 /L to reduce possible septicaemia.[103]
- The haemato-oncologist may also advise granulocyte colony-stimulating factor (G-CSF) prior to dental procedures. One week after the last dose of G-CSF is usually the most appropriate time for dental treatment.

- Local application of tranexamic acid, if available, should be considered, the patient is asked to bite on gauze soaked in tranexamic acid for 15–20 minutes to act as a local antifibrinolytic agent.

- In the event of needing conscious sedation, lymphoma patients require careful assessment as they could be anaemic; conscious sedation should not usually be carried out when the haemoglobin level is less than 10g/dL.36

- Chemotherapy-related mucositis is one of the most common complications following chemotherapy. It affects mucosal areas, including oral mucosa and gastrointestinal tract, and can compromise oral intake. Ice-chips for 30 minutes prior to chemotherapy cycles can help reduce the severity of the developing mucositis.

- Advise patients to follow a soft diet and avoid rough and spicy food, acidic fruit and salt. In severe cases, tube feeding may have to be considered.

- It is important to discuss avoiding smoking and alcohol as this can increase the severity of mucositis.

- Where good oral hygiene is difficult to maintain due to mucositis, a soft toothbrush or sponge toothbrush with alcohol-free mouth rinse can be used.

- Topical gel (lidocaine) or 15% of benzydamine hydrochloride (15 ml three times per day during the chemotherapy cycles) may be prescribed to reduce discomfort and pain.

- Oral infections can present more commonly in patients on chemotherapy due to their immunosuppressed state.

- To prevent fungal infections (eg oral candidiasis), topical anti-fungal agents (ie Nystatin suspension 100,000 U/ml) may be prescribed 4 times per day for 2 weeks.

- Viral infections are also common (mainly herpes simplex), and anti-viral agents may be prescribed (200 mg aciclovir three times per day).

- Both anti-viral and antifungal agents are usually prescribed by the haemato- oncology team as prophylaxis to reduce the development of candidal and viral infections.

DENTAL RECOMMENDATIONS FOR PATIENT UNDERGOING RADIOTHERAPY TREATMENT

- The toxicity associated effects of radiotherapy could be divided into early forms toxicity, such as mucositis, taste disturbance, xerostomia and trismus, or late forms of toxicity, such as irradiation caries and osteoradionecrosis (ORN).

- Patients are expected to have mild acute side-effects, such as dry mouth, mucositis and loss of taste, with low risk of developing ORN.

- It is advisable that patients have a pre-treatment dental assessment. The aim of this assessment is to eliminate any foci of infection, extract poor prognosis teeth, and carry out supragingival and subgingival scaling.

- For dry mouth, patients could take sips of water frequently, and use sugar-free chewing gum to stimulate unaffected salivary cells.The natural mucin-based saliva substitute (AS Pharma Saliva Orthana) and Biotene® Oral Balance Moisturizing Gel or Spray (GlaxoSmith Kline, Brentford) could be prescribed to help reduce the feeling of dryness and lubricate the oral cavity.

- Difflam (15% benzydamine oral rinse, 15 ml every 8 hours and up to 3 weeks post-radiotherapy treatment) is usually prescribed by the patient's haemato- oncology team and acts effectively as an analgesic and antiinflammatory for oral mucositis.

DENTAL RECOMMENDATIONS FOR PATIENTS UNDERGOING CORTICOSTEROID TREATMENT

- A serious oral complication can develop following treatment with bisphosphonate called bisphosphonate-related osteonecrosis of the jaw (BRONJ).

- A dental assessment by the dentist prior to starting the therapy with a drug with a risk of MRONJ is recommended to ensure that patients are dentally fit. This may involve extraction of infected or unrestorable teeth, or teeth with advanced periodontal disease. This should be carried out as soon as possible, and in liaison with a special care dentist or oral surgeon and the haemato-oncologist.

- Dental procedures can increase patient anxiety, which theoretically could lead to adrenal crisis.

- Steroid supplement is not recommended for non-invasive dental procedures (restorative treatment, root canal treatment, supragingival and subgingival scaling).

- For surgical dental procedures under local anaesthesia, steroid supplement is sometimes advised. A double dose of prednisolone or equivalent is recommended one hour before dental treatment, up to a maximum dose of 20 mg hydrocortisone (or equivalent glucocorticoid) or intravenous hydrocortisone may be given. However, steroid cover is assessed case by case and with liaison with a patient's haemato-oncology team.

DENTAL RECOMMENDATIOND FOR PATIENTS UNDERGOING HAEMATOPOIETIC STEM CELL TRANSPLANTATION TREATMENT

- Prior to haematopoietic stem cell transplant (HSCT), patients have reduced platelets and neutrophils due to a high dose of chemotherapy received in preparation for the transplant. This will increase the risk of bleeding episodes and infection. Therefore, pre-treatment dental assessment for patients undergoing HSCT is crucial to eliminate any foci of infection.

- Extraction of teeth with poor prognosis and supragingival and subgingival scaling is recommended, liaison with the haemato-oncology at this stage prior to dental treatment is important.

- A minimum of 10–14 days is recommended for healing after extraction prior to the start of chemotherapy to prevent serious infections while a patient is very immunocompromised.

- Patients with platelet counts below 50 x 109 /L and neutrophil counts below 2 x 109 /L may need pre-operative platelet transfusions and G-CSF plus antibiotic cover to prevent post-operative infections. These patients are better managed in a secondary care centre.

- During the first six months following HSCT, elective dental treatment is not recommended. Where possible, urgent dental problems are better managed through tooth extirpation and/or antibiotics and should be carried out at a secondary care centre.

- Six months post-HSCT, patients can be discharged to primary care for routine follow-up and dental treatment.

- General dental practitioners are advised to consult with a patient's haemato- oncology team or general physician (GP) regarding platelet and neutrophil counts prior to invasive dental treatment.

- Ciclosporin affects oral and dental health negatively and leads to gingival hyperplasia. Gingival enlargement complicates oral hygiene, may lead to halitosis, and can also affect oral function.

- Severe cases of gingival enlargement may need a surgical gingivectomy. This will require a multidisciplinary approach with a periodontologist and the haemato-oncology team.

- Post-HSCT, patients are more susceptible to oral infections similar to infections developed during chemotherapy and therefore may require prescription of anti-viral and anti-fungal agents.

- <u>DENTAL COMPLICATIONS</u>

DUE TO CHEMOTHERAPY

- Mouth sores (oral mucositis)
- Bleeding in the mouth

- Dry mouth (xerostomia)/salivary gland dysfunction.
- Tooth decay and gum disease
- Infection
- Pain
- Difficulty swallowing (dysphagia)
- Changes in taste
- Neurotoxicity
- Changes in dental growth and development occur in children.
- Malnutrition or dehydration

DUE TO RADIATION TO THE HEAD AND NECK.

- Breakdown of tissue, bone or muscle in the area receiving radiation
- Tooth decay and gum disease
- Mouth sores (oral mucositis)
- Infection
- Pain
- Dry mouth (xerostomia)/salivary gland dysfunction
- Difficulty swallowing (dysphagia)
- Changes in taste

- Changes in dental growth and development occur in children.
- Malnutrition or dehydration

DUE TO STEM CELL TRANSPLANT.

Patients who receive an allogeneic stem cell transplant have an increased risk of graft- versus-host disease (GVHD). GVHD occurs when transplanted donor cells attack the patient's body. Symptoms of oral GVHD include:

- Mouth sores that are red and ulcerated
- Dry mouth due to a decrease in saliva flow
- Pain from spices, alcohol, or other flavorings
- Problems swallowing
- Change in taste
- Tightness in the skin or in the lining of the mouth

DUE TO BONE-MODIFYING DRUGS.

Bisphosphonates are a class of drugs that prevent bone loss. Patients should understand that although bisphosphonates are effective, these drugs also carry risk to their dental health. Bisphosphonate treatment can cause a rare but serious side effect called "osteonecrosis of the jaw (ONJ)." ONJ causes part of the jaw bone to die, which can lead to pain, open sores and higher risk of tooth loss and infection. Patients should have a dental check-up before starting treatment with this class of drugs and address any dental problems before treatment begins. Doctors will stop the bisphosphonate treatment if ONJ occurs.[102]

C. CNS AND MISCELLANEOUS INTRACRANIAL &INTRASPINAL NEOPLASMS

- INTRODUCTION
- ETIOLOGY
- PATHOPHYSIOLOGY
- CLASSIFICATION
- ORAL MANIFESTATIONS
- DENTAL MANAGEMENT
- DENTAL COMPLICATIONS

• INTRODUCTION

Central nervous system (CNS) tumors include both nonmalignant and malignant tumors of the brain and spinal cord. Primary malignant CNS tumors are the second most common childhood malignancies after hematologic malignancies and are the most common pediatric solid organ tumor.[104] They are the leading cause of morbidity and mortality associated with cancer. Although it affects all ages, the incidence peaks among children between the ages of 3 and 7. In adults and older children, most tumours are supratentorial in location while in young children they are more commonly infratentorial in location.[105]

The incidence of childhood CNS tumor varies from 1.12 to 5.14 cases per 100,000 individuals. Based upon data from the Central Brain Tumor Registry of the United States (CBTRUS), the estimated incidence of primary non-malignant and malignant CNS tumors for children and adolescents up to 19 years of age was 7.18 cases per 100,000 person-year in 2016.[106] More than 100 different histological subtypes of CNS tumors are recognized but their incidence varies with age. Incidence in Africa is around 11 per 10,00,000 and in Japan and Europe it ranges from 20 to 30 per 1,000,000. The male to female ratio is 1.25:1, as slightly higher frequency of medulloblastoma and CNS germinoma is seen in boys.[107]

• ETIOLOGY AND PATHOGENESIS

Development of brain tumors occurs as a consequence of cellular genetic alterations that allow them to evade normal regulatory mechanisms and destruction by the immune system. These changes may be caused by an inherited or acquired (chemical, physical or biological neuro-carcinogens) cause. Overall, only a very small percentage of brain tumors can be ascribed to the effect of inherited inclination. The different environmental factors involved and alleged typically involve ionizing radiation, non- ionizing radiation, N-nitroso compounds, viral infections (JC virus, cytomegalovirus, HIV, SV-40, varicella-zoster, chicken pox) and head injury.[108]

Syndrome	Gene locus	Gene	Type of CNS tumour
NF type 1	17q11	NF1	Neurofibroma, meningioma, optic nerve glioma
NF2	22q12	NF2	Meningioma, schwannoma
TS	9q34, 16p13	TSc1/TSC2	SEGA
VHL	3p35	VHL	Haemangioblastoma
Li-Fraumani	17q13	p53	Glioma
Gorlin's syndrome	9q31		PNET

- <u>CLASSIFICATION</u>

ASTROCYTIC TUMORS

- Subependymal giant cell astrocytoma
- Pilocytic astrocytoma
- Pilomyxoid astrocytoma
- Diffuse astrocytoma

- Pleomorphic xanthoastrocytoma
- Anaplastic astrocytoma
- Glioblastoma
- Giant cell glioblastoma
- Gliosarcoma

OLIGODENDROGLIAL TUMORS

- Oligodendroglioma
- Anaplastic oligodendroglioma

OLIGOASTROCYTIC TUMORS

- Oligoastrocytoma
- Anaplastic oligoastrocytoma

EPENDYMAL TUMORS

- Subependymoma
- Myxopapillary ependymoma
- Ependymoma
- Anaplastic epedymoma

CHOROID PLEXUS TUMORS

- Choroid plexus papilloma
- Atypical choroid plexus papilloma
- Choroid plexus carcinoma

OTHER NEUROEPITHELIAL TUMORS

- Astroblastoma
- Angiocentric glioma
- Chordoid glioma of the third ventricle

NEURONAL AND MIXED NEURONAL-GLIAL TUMORS

- Gangliocytoma
- Ganglioglioma
- Anplastic ganglioglioma
- Desmoplastic infantile astrocytoma and ganglioglioma
- Dysembryplastic neuroepithelial tumor
- Central neurocytoma
- Extraventricular neurocytoma

- Cerebellar liponeurocytoma
- Paraganglioma of the spinal cord
- Papillary glioneuronal tumor
- Rosette-forming glioneuronal tumor of the fourth ventricle

PINEAL TUMORS

- Pineocytoma
- Pineal parenchymal tumor of intermediate differentiation
- Pineoblastoma
- Papillary tumor of the pineal region

EMBRYONAL TUMORS

- Medulloblastoma
- Cns primitive neuroectodermal tumors
- Atypical teratoid/rhabdoid tumor

TUMORS OF CRANIAL AND PARASPINAL NERVES

- Schwannoma
- Neurofibroma

- Perineuroma
- Malignant peripheral nerve sheath tumors

MENINGEAL TUMORS

- Tumors of meningothelial cells
- Mesenchymal tumors
- Primary melanocytic lesions
- Other neoplasms related to the meninges
- Hemangioblastoma

LYMPHOMA AND HEMATOPOIETIC NEOPLASMS

- Malignant lymphoma
- Plasmacytoma
- Granulocytic sarcoma

GERM CELL TUMORS

- Germinoma
- Embryonal carcinoma
- Yolk-sac tumors

- Choriocarcinoma
- Teratoma
- Mixed germ cell tumor

TUMORS OF THE SELLAR REGION

- Craniopharyngioma
- Granular cell tumor of the neurohypophysis
- Pituicytoma
- Spindle cell oncocytoma of the adenohypophysis

METASTATIC TUMORS

- Modified from the WHO Classification of Tumors of the CNS, 2007.[109]

- **ORAL MANIFESTATIONS**

Patients may have one or more of the following osseous, oral and dental features:

- Short maxilla or mandible or cranial base,
- Macrocephaly,
- Low face height,
- Enlargement of the mandibular canal,

- More frequent class III dental malocclusions,
- Alterations in the temporomandibular joint,
- Gingival enlargement,
- High scores of plaque and bleeding indices are often present, as well as an increased clinical attachment loss is high
- Gingiva pigmentation,
- Macroglossia,
- Enlargement of fungiform papillae,
- Impacted, supernumerary, missing, or displaced teeth and
- Periapical cementum dysplasia.[110]

- **DENTAL MANAGEMENT**
  - The patient received instructions on oral care and dental healthy diet.
  - Restoration of carious teeth carious teeth.
  - Antibiotic prohylactic regimen
  - Scaling and root planning
  - Extractions of the infra-occlused primary molars

- **DENTAL COMPLICATIONS**

Owing to the bleeding risk inherent to extractions of the infraocclused primary molars and the fibroid site on left maxillar, various precautions were taken. Local anesthesia of the extraction sites allowed local vasoconstriction. The surgical procedure was the minimally invasive. After completion of the avulsions, haemostatic sponges were placed in the alveolar sockets and we performed sutures using a 3-0 vicryl suture. At the end of the procedure, the hemostasis was checked after local compression.

D. TUMORS OF SYMPATHETIC NERVOUS SYSTEM

- INTRODUCTION
- ETIOLOGY
- PATHOPHYSIOLOGY
- CLASSIFICATION
- ORAL MANIFESTATIONS
- DENTAL MANAGEMENT
- DENTAL COMPLICATIONS

- **INTRODUCTION**

Many reports of tumors arising within the sympathetic nervous system have appeared during the past few years. Many of the tumors were described early. Virchow, in 1864, described an undoubted tumor of the sympathetic system, designating it a glioma. Wright, in 1910, gave one of the best descriptions of one variety of these tumors, such a one as was described by Virchow, and placed these on a sound pathologic basis. The paragangliomas or chromaffin tumors were first described by Manasse in the suprarenal gland in 1893. Frankel (1886) and Perley (1890) apparently described tumors of this type. The third type, ganglioneuromas, were first described by Loretz in 1870. The literature on these tumors has been reviewed several times during recent years. The number of cases studied by any one person has been relatively small.

- **ETIOLOGY & PATHOPHYSIOLOGY**

In the sympathetic nervous system three different types of tumors may arise: neuroblastoma, ganglioneuroma and phaeochromocytoma. All three originate from the same embryonic tissue and have the same anatomical sites. They vary in histology and in cytogenetics but have similar biochemistry. Their symptoms differ, and they are diagnosed and treated by different methods.

After fertilization an ovum passes through the morula and blastula stages; the first signs of development of the central nervous system appear in the gastrula stage. The neural plate, which consists of ectodermal cells, forms in what is referred to as the neurula stage. The margins of the neural plate are elevated to create the neural folds, which are separated by a midline neural groove. With further growth, progressive fusion between the folds takes place. In this way the neural tube is formed, and the connection to the ectoderm disappears. During separation of the neural tube a chain of cells appears on either side in the angle between the tube and the remaining ectoderm. These two longitudinal columns form the neural crest.

From the distal part of the neural crest, cells begin to migrate. The dorsally migrating cells are partially responsible for formation of the melanoblasts. The ventrally migrating cells develop into the spinal ganglia, the ganglia of the sympathetic side chain, the pre-vertebral ganglia, the paraganglia and the chromaffin bodies as well as APUD cells and the leptomeninges. The cells migrating from the neural crest, which form the sympathetic nervous system, are called sympathetic neuroblasts, primitive sympathetic cells or sympathogonia. The sympathogonia migrate further to the adrenal medulla and the paraganglia of Zuckerkandl at the bifurcation of the aorta.

A large number of paraganglia are formed in the retroperitoneal space along the aorta. The sympathogonia are still pluripotential cells at this stage and differentiate into chromaffin cells, neurofibrous cells and ganglion cells. This differentiation starts in the fetus at 10 weeks and continues until long after birth, going on in the adrenal medulla well into adulthood. Apart from the sympathetic side chain, which forms at an early stage of development, sympathetic plexuses, such as the coeliac, mesenteric and renal plexuses, are formed. In adults these consist of ganglion cells and sporadic chromaffin cells. In the fetus and newborn the cell morphology is found to vary widely. The

paraganglia are also important at this age, both anatomically and endocrinologically. At 2-3 years of age the adrenal medulla is well developed, and the paraganglia are in decline. When the sympathetic tissue is still immature sympathogonia, either in mitosis or not, all intermediate stages of differentiation to chromaffin cells, neurofibrous cells and ganglion cells are found side by side. This variety can make a precise diagnosis difficult when a tumor arises in the sympathetic nervous system.

- **<u>CLASSIFICATION</u>**

  - Neuroblastoma,

- Ganglioneuroma and
- Phaeochromocytoma.

- **<u>ORAL MANIFESTATIONS</u>**
  - Facial swelling,
  - Intraoral masses,
  - Loose or displaced teeth, and
  - Alterations in nerve function
  - Sudden neurological changes as indicated by pain or numbness. These alterations were apparently related to tumor invasion in the area of the inferior alveolar nerve.
  - Radiographic evidence of oral metastasis such as ill-defined borders around the crypts of developing teeth, expansion of the dental follicle, displaced or floating teeth or both, and lytic lesions.
  - Loss of definition of the white borders around dental crypts was seen.
  - Unilateral or bilateral expansion of the dental follicle with displacement of the tooth bud was seen.
  - The absence of supporting bone around these teeth sometimes suggested the appearance of floating teeth.
  - Lytic lesions, the most common pathologic change. The lesions were confined to the posterior body and ramus area of the mandible, and their appearances ranged from a decreased area of density to irregular lucent areas with complete dissolution of the osseous architecture. Although the lesions destroyed bone and moved teeth, they did not resorb the roots of teeth. Sclerotic borders, reactive bone, and periosteal reactions were not seen.

- **DENTAL MANAGEMENT & COMPLICATIONS**

  - Identify and stabilize or eliminate existing and potential sources of infection and local irritants in the oral cavity.

  - Communicate with the medical team regarding the patient's oral health status, plan, and timing of treatment.

  - Educate the patient and parents about the importance of optimal oral care to minimize oral problems and discomfort.

  - Medical history review should include disease/condition (type, stage, prognosis), treatment protocol (conditioning regimen, surgery, chemotherapy, location and dose of radiation), medications (including bisphosphonates and other bone modifying agents), allergies, surgeries, secondary medical diagnoses, hematological status (e.g. Complete blood count [cbc]), immunosuppression status, presence of an indwelling venous access line, and contact of medical team/primary care physician(s).

  - Oral hygiene: brushing of the teeth and tongue two to three times daily should be performed with a regular soft nylon-bristled or electric toothbrush, regardless of hematological status. Ultrasonic brushes and dental floss should only be allowed if the patient is properly trained. If capable, the patient's teeth should be gently flossed daily. If pain or excessive bleeding occurs, the patient should avoid the affected area, but floss the other teeth. Patients with poor oral hygiene and/or periodontal disease may use chlorhexidine rinses until the tissue health improves or mucositis develops. The high alcohol content of commercially available chlorhexidine mouthwash may cause discomfort and dehydrate the tissues in patients with mucositis. An alcohol-free chlorhexidine solution is indicated in this situation.
  - Dental practitioners should discuss the importance of a healthy diet to maintain nutritional status and emphasize food choices that do not promote caries.

Patients and parents should be advised about the high cariogenic potential of carbohydrate-rich dietary supplements and sucrose-sweetened medications.

- Preventive measures include the use of fluoridated toothpaste, fluoride supplements if indicated, neutral fluoride gels/rinses, or applications of fluoride varnish for patients at risk for caries and/or dry mouth. A brush-on technique is convenient and may increase the likelihood of patient compliance with topical fluoride therapy.

- Dental providers should be aware of the patient's hematologic status and related risks of bacteremia and excessive bleeding. Hematologic management of the patient should be directed by the patient's oncologist, and consultation with the medical team is necessary to determine the need for prophylactic interventions prior to dental treatment. A decision regarding the need for antibiotic prophylaxis prior to dental treatment should be made in consultation with the child's physician.[111]

References

1. Costa, L. S.; Côrrea, M. S. N. P.; Imparato, J. C. P.; Rezende, K. M. Overview Of Oral Manifestations Resulting From The Treatment Of Childhood Cancer: An Integrative Review. Research, Society And Development, *[S. L.]*, V. 10, N. 8, P.
2. IARC Press release, 2013. Available from http://ci5.iarc.fr/ [Accessed on May 02, 2014].
3. Rebecca L. Siegel, Kimberly D. Miller, Ahmedin Jemal. Cancer Statistics. Ca Cancer J Clin. 2020; (0):1–24.
4. Cabrerizo-Merino, C., & Onate-Sanchez, R.E. (2005). Some odontostomatological aspects in childhood oncology. Medicina Oral, Patologia Oral y Cirugia Bucal [Oral Medicine, Oral Pathology, and Oral Surgery], 10, 41–47.
5. Alberth, M., Majoros, L., Kovalecz, G., Borbas, E., Szegedi, I., Marton, I.J., & Kiss, C. (2006). Significance of oral Candida infections in children with cancer. Pathology Oncology Research, 12, 237–241.
6. American Academy of Pediatric Dentistry. (2008). Guidelines on the dental management of pediatric patients receiving chemotherapy, hematopoietic cell transplantation, and/or radiation. Retrieved from http://www.aapd.org/media/Policies_Guidelines/G_Chemo.pdf.
7. Rojas de Morales, T., Zambrano, O., Rivera, L., Navas, R., Chaparro, N., Bernardonni, C., . . . Tirado, D.M. (2001). Oral-disease pre Oral-disease prevention in children with cancer: Testing preventive protocol effectiveness. Medicina Oral [Oral Medicine], 6, 326–234.
8. Gabrielle Allen, Richard Logan, and Sam Gue. Oral Manifestations of Cancer Treatment in Children. Clinical Journal of Oncology Nursing. 2010;14 (4).
9. National Cancer Control Program of India. Available from: http://www.nihfw.org/NationalHealthProgramme/NATIONALCANCERCONTROLPROGRAMME.html.
10. Shetty R, Mathew RT, Vijayakumar M. Incidence and pattern of distribution of cancer in India: A secondary data analysis from six population-based cancer registries. Cancer Res Stat Treat 2020;3:678-82.
11. Globocan2020 India Fact Sheet. Available from: https://gco.iarc.fr/today/data/factsheets/populations/356-india-fact-sheets.pdf.

12. International Incidence of Childhood Cancer. Available from: http://iicc.iarc.fr/results/comparative.php.
13. Atun R, Bhakta N, Denburg A, Frazier AL, Friedrich P, Gupta S, *et al*. Sustainable care for children with cancer: A lancet oncology commission. Lancet Oncol 2020;21:e185-e224.
14. Wolfe A. Institute of Medicine Report: Crossing the Quality Chasm: A New Health Care System for the 21st Century. Policy Polit Nurs Pract 2001;2:233- 5.
15. Infant Mortality Rate in India. Available from: https://www.statista.com/statistics/806931/infant-mortality-in-india/.
16. Arora RS, Eden TOB, Kapoor G. Epidemiology of childhood cancer in India. Indian Journal of Cancer. 2009: 46; 4:3321-5
17. Ries L, Smith M, Gurney JG, et al., editors. Cancer incidence and survival among children and adolescents: United States SEER program 1975-1999 [NIH (Pub. No. 99-4649]. Bethesda (MD): National Cancer Institute, SEER program; 1999. Available from: http://www.seer.cancer.gov.
18. Stiller CA, Parkin DM. Geographic and ethnic variations in the incidence of childhood cancer. Br Med Bull 1996;52:682-703.
19. Gurney JG, Bondy ML. Epidemiology of childhood cancer. In: Pizzo PA, Poplack DG, Editors. Priciples and Practice of Pediatric Oncology, 5th edition. Philadelphia; Lippincott Williams and Wilkins: 2006. P. 2-14.
20. Barr R, Riberio R, Agarwal B, Masera G, Hesseling P, Magrath I. Pediatric Oncology in Countries with Limited Resources. In: Pizzo PA, Poplack DG, eds. Principles and Practice of Pediatric Oncology, 5th ed. Philadelphia: Lippincott Williams and Wilkins; 2006. p. 1605-17.
21. Swaminathan R, Rama R, Shanta V. Childhood cancers in Chennai, India, 1990-2001: incidence and survival. Int J Cancer 2008;122:2607-11.
22. Miller RW. Frequency and environmental epidemiology of childhood cancer. In: Principles and Practice of Pediatric Oncology (Pizzo PA, Poplack DG, eds). Philadelphia:JB Lippincott, 1989;3-18.
23. Stewart AM, Webb J, Hewitt D. A survey of childhood malignancies. Br Med J 1,1958: 1495-1508
24. Tucker MA, D'Angio GJ, Boice JD Jr, Strong LC, Li FP, Stovell M, Stone BJ, Green DM, Lombardi F, Newton W, Hoover RN, Fraumeni JF Jr. Bone sarcomas linked to radiotherapy and chemotherapy in children. N Engl J Med 1987, 317:588-593 .
25. Theriault G. Electromagnetic fields and cancer risks. Rev Epiddm et Sante Publ 1992,40:S55-S62 .

26. Wertheimer N, Leeper E. Electrical wiring configurations and childhood cancer. Am J Epidemiol 1979,109:273-284.
27. James JE. Maternal caffeine consumption and pregnancy outcomes: a narrative review with implications for advice to mothers and mothers-to-be. BMJ Evidence-Based Medicine. 2020.
28. Council on Scientific Affairs,(1983) Fetal effects of maternal alcohol use. JAMA 249:2517-2521 .
29. Goh YI, Bollano E, Einarson TR, Koren G. Prenatal multivitamin supplementation and rates of pediatric cancers: a meta-analysis. Clin Pharmacol Ther. 2007; 81(5):685–91.
30. Melnick S, Cole P, Anderson D, Herbst A.(1987) Rates and risks of diethylstilbestrol related clear-cell adenocarcinoma of the vagina and cervix: an update. N Engl J Med 316:514-516 .
31. Allen RW, Ogden B, Bently FL, Jung AL.(1980) Fetal hydantoin syndrome, neuroblastoma, and hemorrhagic disease in a neonate. JAMA 244:1464-1465
32. Blattner WA, Henson DE, Young RC, Fraumeni JF (1977).Jr. Malignant mesenchymoma and birth defects: prenatal exposure to phenytoin. J Am Med Assoc 238:334-335 .
33. Kramer S, Ward E, Meadows AT, Malone K.(1987).Medical and drug risk factors associated with neuroblastoma: a case-control study. J Natl Cancer Inst 78:797-804 .
34. Lindblad P, Zack M, Adami H-O, Ericson A.(1992). Maternal and perinatal risk factors for Wilms' tumor: a nationwide nested case-control study in Sweden. Int J Cancer 51:38-41 .
35. Grufferman S, Schwartz AG, Ruymann FB, Maurer HM.(1993). Parents' use of cocaine and marijuana and increased risk of rhabdomyosarcoma in their children. Cancer Causes Control 4:217-224 .
36. Robison LL, Buckley J, Daigle A, Arthur DC, Wells R, Benjamin D, Hammond GD.(1989) Maternal drug use and risk of a childhood non-lymphoblastic leukemia among offspring: a report from the Children's Cancer Study Group. Cancer 64:1169-1176 .
37. Kuijten RR, Bunin GR, Nass CC, Meadows AT. (1990). Gestational and familial risk factors for childhood astrocytoma: results of a case-control study. Cancer Res 50:2608-2612.
38. Grufferman S, Wang HH, DeLong ER, Kimm SYS, Delzell ES, Falletta JM.(1982). Environmental factors in the etiology of rhabdomyosarcoma in childhood. J Natl Cancer Inst 68:107-113 .

39. Infante PF, Newton WA.(1975). Prenatal chlordane exposure and neuroblastoma. N Engl J Med 293:308 .
40. Reeves JD, Driggers DA, Kiley VA. (1981); Household insecticide associated aplastic anaemia and acute leukaemia in children. Lancet 8241:300.
41. Wagner JC, Sleggs CA, Marchand P.(1960); Diffuse pleural mesothelioma and asbestos exposure in the North Western Cape Province. Br J Ind Med 17:260-271 .
42. Stewart PA, Herrick RF.(1991); Issues in performing retrospective exposure assessment. Apple Occup Environ Hyg 6:421-427 .
43. Morrow RH Jr. Burkitt's lymphoma. In: Cancer Epidemiology and Prevention (Schottenfeld D, Fraumeni JF Jr, eds). Philadelphia:WB Saunders, 1982;779- 794.
44. Milne E, Greenop KR, Metayer C, Schuz J, Petridou E, Pombo-de-Oliveira MS, et al. Fetal growth and childhood acute lymphoblastic leukemia: findings from the childhood leukemia international consortium. Int J Cancer. 2013; 133(12):2968–79.
45. Johnson KJ, Carozza SE, Chow EJ, Fox EE, Horel S, McLaughlin CC, et al. Parental age and risk of childhood cancer: a pooled analysis. Epidemiology. 2009; 20(4):475–83.
46. Botto LD, Flood T, Little J, Fluchel MN, Krikov S, Feldkamp ML, et al. Cancer risk in children and adolescents with birth defects: a population-based cohort study. PLoS One. 2013; 8(7):e69077.
47. Seif AE. Pediatric leukemia predisposition syndromes: clues to understanding leukemogenesis. Cancer Genet. 2011; 204(5):227–44.
48. Choong SS, Latiff ZA, Mohamed M, Lim LL, Chen KS, Vengidasan L, et al. Childhood adrenocortical carcinoma as a sentinel cancer for detecting families with germline TP53 mutations. Clin Genet. 2012; 82(6):564–8.
49. Viswanath D, Umashankar DN, Kumar MR. Common Paediatric Malignancies: a Review. J Indian Aca Oral Med Radiol 2013;25(2):0-0.
50. Pfister SM, Reyes-Múgica M, Chan JKC, Hasle H, Lazar AJ, Rossi S, Ferrari A, Jarzembowski JA, Pritchard-Jones K, Hill DA, Jacques TS, Wesseling P, López Terrada DH, von Deimling A, Kratz CP, Cree IA, Alaggio R. A Summary of the Inaugural WHO Classification of Pediatric Tumors: Transitioning from the Optical into the Molecular Era. Cancer Discov. 2022 Feb;12(2):331-355.
51. Metayer C, Dahl G, Wiemels J, Miller M. Childhood Leukemia: A Preventable Disease. Pediatrics. 2016 Nov;138(Suppl 1):S45-S55. doi:

10.1542/peds.2015-4268H. PMID: 27940977; PMCID: PMC5080868.
52. Stieglitz, E.; Loh, M.L. Genetic predispositions to childhood leukemia. Ther. Adv. Hematol. 2013, 4, 270–290.
53. Tebbi, C.K. Etiology of Acute Leukemia: A Review. Cancers 2021, 13, 2256.
54. Brown, W.C.; Doll, R.; Hill, A.B. Incidence of leukaemia after exposure to diagnostic radiation in utero. Br. Med. J. 1960, 2, 1539.
55. Stewart, A.; Webb, J.; Giles, D.; Hewitt, D. Malignant disease in childhood and diagnostic irradiation in utero. Lancet 1956, 268, 447.
56. Kleinerman, R.A. Cancer risks following diagnostic and therapeutic radiation exposure in children. Pediatr. Radiol. 2006, 36, 121–125.
57. Gardner, M.J. Review of reported increases of childhood cancer rates in the vicinity of nuclear installations in the UK. J. R. Stat. Soc. Ser. A 1989, 152, 307–325.
58. Meinert, R.; Kaletsch, U.; Kaatsch, P.; Schüz, J.; Michaelis, J. Associations between childhood cancer and ionizing radiation: Results of a population-based case-control study in Germany. Cancer Epidemiol. Prev. Biomark. 1999, 8, 793–799.
59. Bhatia, S.; Robison, L.L. Epidemiology of leukemia and lymphoma. Curr. Opin. Hematol. 1999, 6, 201.
60. Blair, A.; Zheng, T.; Linos, A.; Stewart, P.A.; Zhang, Y.W.; Cantor, K.P. Occupation and leukemia: A population-based case-control study in Iowa and Minnesota. Am. J. Ind Med. 2001, 40, 3–14.
61. Wong, O.; Harris, F.; Armstrong, T.W.; Hua, F. A hospital-based case-control study of acute myeloid leukemia in Shanghai: Analysis of environmental and occupational risk factors by subtypes of the WHO classification. Chem. Biol. Interact. 2010, 184, 112–128.
62. Finch, S.C. Radiation-induced leukemia: Lessons from history. Best Pract. Res. Clin. Haematol. 2007, 20, 109–118.
63. Beane Freeman, L.E.; Deroos, A.J.; Koutros, S.; Blair, A.; Ward, M.H.; Alavanja, M.; Hoppin, J.A. Poultry and livestock exposure and cancer risk among farmers in the agricultural health study. Cancer Causes Control. 2012, 23, 663–670.
64. Moloney, W.C. Leukemia in survivors of atomic bombing. N. Engl. J. Med. 1955, 253, 88–90. .
65. Kleinerman, R.A.; Kaune, W.T.; Hatch, E.E.; Wacholder, S.; Linet, M.S.; Robison, L.L.; Niwa, S.; Tarone, R.E. Are children living near high-voltage power lines at increased risk of acute lymphoblastic leukemia? Am. J.

Epidemiol. 2000, 151, 512–515.
66. Infante-Rivard, C.; Deadman, J.E. Maternal occupational exposure to extremely low frequency magnetic fields during pregnancy and childhood leukemia. Epidemiology 2003, 14, 437–441.
67. Tebbi, C.K.; London, W.B.; Friedman, D.; Villaluna, D.; De Alarcon, P.A.; Constine, L.S.; Mendenhall, N.P.; Sposto, R.; Chauvenet, A.; Schwartz, C.L. Dexrazoxane-associated risk for acute myeloid leukemia/myelodysplastic syndrome and other secondary malignancies in pediatric Hodgkin's disease. J. Clin. Oncol. 2007, 25, 493–500.
68. Lin, C.K.; Hsu, Y.T.; Brown, K.D.; Pokharel, B.; Wei, Y.; Chen, S.T. Residential exposure to petrochemical industrial complexes and the risk of leukemia: A systematic review and exposure-response meta-analysis. Environ. Pollut. 2020, 258, 113476.
69. Menegaux, F.; Baruchel, A.; Bertrand, Y.; Lescoeur, B.; Leverger, G.; Nelken, B.; Sommelet, D.; Hémon, D.; Clavel, J. Household exposure to pesticides and risk of childhood acute leukaemia. Occup. Environ. Med. 2006, 63, 131–134.
70. Knox, E. Childhood cancers and atmospheric carcinogens. J. Epidemiol. Community Health 2005, 59, 101–105.
71. Reigstad, M.M.; Larsen, I.K.; Myklebust, T.Å.; Robsahm, T.E.; Oldereid, N.B.; Brinton, L.A.; Storeng, R. Risk of Cancer in Children Conceived by Assisted Reproductive Technology. Pediatrics 2016, 137, e20152061.
72. Pang, D.; McNally, R.; Birch, J.M. Parental smoking and childhood cancer: Results from the United Kingdom Childhood Cancer Study. Br. J. Cancer 2003, 88, 373–381.
73. Robison, L.L.; Buckley, J.D.; Daigle, A.E.; Wells, R.; Benjamin, D.; Arthur, D.C.; Hammond, G.D. Maternal drug use and risk of childhood nonlymphoblastic leukemia among offspring. An epidemiologic investigation implicating marijuana (a report from the Childrens Cancer Study Group). Cancer 1989, 63, 1904–1911.
74. Dockerty, J.D.; Draper, G.; Vincent, T.; Rowan, S.D.; Bunch, K.J. Case-control study of parental age, parity and socioeconomic level in relation to childhood cancers. Int. J. Epidemiol. 2001, 30, 1428–1437.
75. Tebbi, C.K.; Badiga, A.; Sahakian, E.; Arora, A.I.; Nair, S.; Powers, J.J.; Achille, A.N.; Jaglal, M.V.; Patel, S.; Migone, F. Plasma of Acute Lymphoblastic Leukemia Patients React to the Culture of a Mycovirus Containing Aspergillus Flavus. J. Pediatr. Hematol. Oncol. 2020, 42, 350–358.

76. Chabay, P.A.; Preciado, M.V. EBV primary infection in childhood and its relation to B-cell lymphoma development: A mini-review from a developing region. Int. J. Cancer 2013, 133, 1286–1292.
77. Daniel A. Arber, Attilio Orazi, Robert Hasserjian, Jürgen Thiele, Michael J. Borowitz, Michelle M. Le Beau, Clara D. Bloomfield, Mario Cazzola, James W. Vardiman. The 2016 revision to the World Health Organization classification of myeloid neoplasms and acute leukemia. *Blood* (2016) 127 (20): 2391–2405.
78. Dean A, Ferguson J, Marvanr E (2003). Acute leukaemia presenting as oral ulceration to a dental emergency service. Australian Dental J, 48, 195-7.
79. Hou GL, Huang JS, Tsai CC (1997). Analysis of oral manifestations of leukemia: a retrospective study. Oral Dis, 3, 31-8.
80. Auluck A, Zhang L, Desai R, et al (2008). Primary malignant melanoma of maxillary gingiva--a case report and review of the literature. J Can Dent Assoc, 74, 367-71.
81. da Silva Santos PS, Fontes A, de Andrade F, et al (2010). Gingival leukemic infiltration as the first manifestation of acute myeloid leukemia. Otolaryngol Head Neck Surgery, 143, 465-6.
82. Declerck D, Vinckier F (1988). Oral complications of leukemia. Quintessence Int, 19, 575-83.
83. Aronovich S, Connolly TW (2008). Pericoronitis as an initial manifestation of acute lymphoblastic leukemia: a case report. J Oral and Maxillofacial Surgery, 66, 804-8.
84. Katz J, Peretz B (2002). Trismus in a 6 year old child: a manifestation of leukemia? Journal of Clinical Pediatric Dentistry, 26, 337-9.
85. Anirudhan D, Bakhshi S, Xess I, et al (2008). Etiology and outcome of oral mucosal lesions in children on chemotherapy for acute lymphoblastic leukemia. Indian Pediatr, 45, 47-51.
86. Caroline Zimmermann,1 Maria Inês Meurer,2,3 Liliane Janete Grando,2,3 Joanita Ângela Gonzaga Del Moral,4 Inês Beatriz da Silva Rath,5 and Silvia Schaefer Tavares6. Dental Treatment in Patients with Leukemia. Journal of Oncology. 2015;
87. J. W. Little, D. A. Falace, C. S. Miller, and N. L. Rhodus, "Disorders of white blood cells," in Dental Magenement of the Medically Compromised Patient, pp. 373–395, 2007.
88. American Academy of Pediatric Dentistry, "Guideline on dental management of pediatric patients receiving chemotherapy,

hematopoietic cell transplantation, and/or radiation," Journal of Pediatric Dentistry, vol. 35, no. 5, pp. E185–E193, 2013, http://www.ncbi.nlm.nih.gov/pubmed/24290549.

89. Lowal KA, Alaizari NA, Tarakji B, Petro W, Hussain KA, Altamimi MA. DENTAL CONSIDERATIONS FOR LEUKEMIC PEDIATRIC PATIENTS: AN UPDATED REVIEW FOR GENERAL DENTAL PRACTITIONER. Mater Sociomed. 2015 Oct;27(5):359-62. doi: 10.5455/msm.2015.27.359-362. Epub 2015 Oct 5. PMID: 26622207; PMCID: PMC4639337.
90. Morais EF, Lira JA, Macedo RA, Santos KS, Elias CT, Morais Mde L. Oral manifestations resulting from chemotherapy in children with acute lymphoblastic leukemia. *Braz J Otorhinolaryngol.* 2014;80:78–85.
91. Dholam KP, Gurav S, Dugad J, Banavli S. Correlation of oral health of children with acute leukemia during the induction phase. *Indian J Med Paediatr Oncol.* 2014;35:36–39.
92. Martin PJ, Weisdorf D, Przepiorka D, Hirschfeld S, Farrell A, Rizzo JD, et al. Design of Clinical Trials Working Group. National Institutes of Health Consensus Development Project on Criteria for Clinical Trials in Chronic Graft-versus-Host Disease: VI. Design of Clinical Trials Working Group report. *Biol Blood Marrow Transplant.* 2006;5:491–505.
93. de Oliveira Lula EC, de Oliveira Lula CE, Alves CM, Lopes FF, Pereira AL. Chemotherapy-induced oral complications in leukemic patients. *Int J Pediatr Otorhinolaryngol.* 2007;71:1681–1685.
94. Allen CE, Kelly KM, Bollard CM. Pediatric lymphomas and histiocytic disorders of childhood. Pediatr Clin North Am. 2015 Feb;62(1):139-65. doi: 10.1016/j.pcl.2014.09.010. PMID: 25435117; PMCID: PMC4250829.
95. National Cancer Institute Physician Data Query (PDQ). Childhood Non-Hodgkin Lymphoma Treatment. 2021. Accessed at https://www.cancer.gov/types/lymphoma/patient/child-nhl-treatment-pdq on June 10, 2021.
96. De Leval, L., & Jaffe, E. S. (2020). *Lymphoma Classification. The Cancer Journal, 26(3), 176–185.*
97. . Silva TDB, Belo C, Ferreira T, Leite GB, Roberto J, Pontes DM, et al. Oral manifestations of lymphoma : a systematic review. Ecancermedicalscience. 2016;10:665.
98. Alexiev BA, Sailey CJ, McClure SA, Ord RA, Zhao XF, Papadimitriou JC. Primary Zhistiocytic sarcoma arising in the head and neck with predominant spindle cell component. Diagn Pathol. 2007;2:7.

99. Bassuner J, Miranda RN, Emge DA, Dicicco BA, Lewis DJ, Duvic M. Mycosis Fungoides of the Oral Cavity: Fungating Tumor Successfully Treated with Electron Beam Radiation and Maintenance Bexarotene. 2016.
100. Davis G, Perks A, Liyanage P. Oral hairy leukoplakia arising in a patient with hairy cell leukemia: the first reported case. BMJ Case Reports. 2017.
101. Abed, H., Nizarali, N., & Burke, M. (2019). *Oral and dental management for people with lymphoma. Dental Update, 46(2), 133–150.*
102. Scully C, Diz Dios P, Kumar N. Special Care in Dentistry. London: Elsevier, 2002 CNS
103. Linabery AM, Ross JA. Trends in childhood cancer incidence in the U.S.(1992-2004). Cancer 2008; 112:416.
104. Raizer J. Faculty of 1000 evaluation for CBTRUS Statistical Report: Primary brain and other central nervous system tumors diagnosed in the United States in 2010-2014. F1000. 2018. Post-publication peer review of the biomedical literature.
105. Ostrom QT, Gittleman H, Xu J, Kromer C, Wolinsky Y, Kruchko C, et al. CBTRUS statistical report: Primary brain and other central nervous system tumors diagnosed in the United States in 2009-2013. Neuro-Oncology. 2016;18:v1-v75.
106. Mckinney PA. Central nervous system tumours in children: Epidemiology and risk factors. Bioelectromagnetics. 2005;26(S7).
107. Santos MM, Faria CC, Miguéns J. Pediatric central nervous system tumors: Review of a single Portuguese institution. Child's Nervous System. 2016;32:1227-1236.
108. Kaatsch P, Rickert CH, Kuhl J, Schuz J, Michaelis J. Population-based epidemiologic data on brain tumors in German children. Cancer. 2001;92:3155-3164.
109. Javed F, Ramalingam S, Ahmed HB, Gupta B, Sundar C, Qadri T. Oral manifestations in patients with neurofibromatosis type-1: a comprehensive literature review. *Crit Rev Oncol Hematol.* 2014;91:123–9.

www.ingramcontent.com/pod-product-compliance
Lightning Source LLC
LaVergne TN
LVHW021252160826
845679LV00001B/47

9798891336643